CONTENTS

INTRODUCTION

Anyone who's ever had a migraine – and you can include me in that – can understand without question the misery it brings.

I've been fortunate, I've only had two attacks. The first was about twenty years ago when I had a classical aura, which you'll read about later if you don't know what I mean. This was followed by a one-sided headache which was unpleasant but nothing more than that.

The second was about fifteen years ago. That one was a real zonker and I'll never forget it. I'd taken two of my three children to an afternoon cinema performance and we'd had to sit quite near to the front. The large screen had seemed rather close and flickery and I'd felt a little disorientated while watching the film. The soundtrack was rather loud, too, I remember.

As we came out I was aware of the shimmering on one side of my vision and now knew exactly what was meant by a 'fortification spectrum'. The shimmering I was experiencing looked like the battlements of a toy fort that I'd had as a child. I expected to get a headache like I'd had before – but not a bit of it. What followed was the worst physical pain I'd ever had in my life. I didn't know where to put myself. Fortunately, I'd got home by this time but I wanted to bash my head against the wall. I ended up lying on the floor of our bedroom. Not the bed. For some reason which I must have had at the time, the floor seemed preferable. Perhaps the discomfort in some way took the horror away from my head.

I'd drawn the curtains, taken a non-recommendably large dose of aspirin but didn't expect to keep it down as I felt so sick. And I didn't! I lay there hoping that *anything* would happen since it would be better than this, when, after what seemed like hours, I must have fallen asleep. When I woke up an hour later the pain had gone. I've never had it again.

So, once you've suffered a migraine headache, or perhaps have lived with someone who suffers from migraine, you'll realise – like me – that it's like no other type of headache and that migraine sufferers deserve more sympathy and understanding than they sometimes receive.

In my experience as a doctor and of answering people's queries on the *Jimmy Young Show* and on my *Woman's Own* letters page, migraine sufferers have continually told me how they are often branded as 'neurotic' and actually made to feel guilty about their 'weakness'.

This guilt complex is completely unfair even if migraine was a weakness. But it's *not* and studies have shown that there is no typical 'migraine personality'. And you shouldn't automatically assume that a migraine sufferer is an anxious, worrying type – even though from time to time I still come across the view that if you're a migraine sufferer you must be sensitive and intelligent. Not that I want to imply that migraine sufferers are neither!

What I do want to stress is that sufferers come from all walks of life, and they have all kinds of personalities and temperaments. Wimps and macho men included! I do feel that it's quite important to get this message across, not only to families, friends and colleagues of migraine sufferers, but also to the sufferers themselves. Making them feel less 'branded' is an important aspect of coming to terms with migraine and of learning how to cope with it. If you suffer from migraine there's nothing 'wrong' with you, you're not sickly or unhealthy, it's just the way your body behaves. Some studies have shown that many migraine sufferers are conscientious, perfectionist, persistent and exacting – and since they're all potentially admirable traits I'm not going to disagree too strongly! However, other researchers say that these characteristics are more likely to be due to bias in the research – and I'm far more inclined towards this view. Summed up this means that I believe migraine sufferers are the same as everyone else, except for this infuriating susceptibility to migraine.

While I think of it, though, there is one thing migraine sufferers do seem to have in common. Time and again I've found that they tend to accept their lot in silence and soldier on with the problem stoically. Some don't like to bother their doctor about their headaches and many don't even like to discuss with anyone the fact that they suffer from the condition – mainly because of the attitudes of people who are fortunately migraine-free. This stems from a genuine fear of being branded a lame duck, a shirker or someone with a low pain threshold, rather than someone who just happens to get migraine. Men are said to be even more reluctant to discuss the problem than women – possibly out of a concern for jeopardising career prospects or for fear of being considered unreliable.

But while it is not possible to cure a migraine sufferer completely, help can be given and it should be possible for most sufferers to find something to help them reduce the frequency of their attacks or lessen their severity. In this book I set out to explain simply what migraine is, what different types exist, what can be done about the condition, either by your GP and the medicines he or she can prescribe for you or the medicines – that's conventional, herbal and homoeopathic – that you can buy for yourself over-the-counter in pharmacies or health shops; I explain the various complementary treatments that may be worth trying and I give advice on self-help measures that could ease your migraine. Some tips I've gleaned over the years and other pieces of practical advice on coping that comes from talking to migraine sufferers themselves. So, if in the past you've felt like giving up hope, please read on.

First, I'd like to point out that in spite of the frequent misunderstanding migraine brings with it, it is, in fact, a very common condition, and not just in modern times. According to the Migraine Trust, which raises funds for research, migraine shares with epilepsy the dark distinction of being one of the two conditions known the longest to practising physicians. Four centuries before Christ, Hippocrates gave excellent accounts of both disorders. Migraine is not without its claim to fame where well-known names are concerned – Julius Caesar, Joan of Arc, Peter the Great of Russia, Richard Wagner and Princess Margaret are all said to have suffered from it.

These days every GP is likely to have anywhere from one hundred to two hundred patients on his or her list who suffer from migraine. It affects as many as one in ten people (mainly women, possibly in the ratio of two women to every man) of any race, occupation, class or age, including children. Other estimates suggest that migraineurs could number as many as one in seven people or that between 6 and 10 million people in Britain could suffer from it. There appears to be no age barrier although it usually seems to affect more people below the age of forty.

Migraine, in the main, does decrease in frequency as a sufferer gets older. This is possibly due to the general loss of elasticity of artery walls that seems to come with the ageing process – though goodness knows if that is really the reason.

Likewise, because more women suffer than men,

female hormones may be responsible, in part. But that is used as a reason for so many minor differences between the sexes that I think it's unlikely to be the total answer.

And yes, it can run in families. I would also go as far as to say that roughly three-quarters of migraine patients have close relatives who have had attacks. Often a patient has a mother with the same problem.

One of the unusual aspects of migraine is that in many ways it's a different thing to different people. For example, frequency can vary greatly, from only once or twice a year to several times a week. The severity and type of symptoms differ widely, too. A sufferer may find that he or she has a mild attack at one time and then a severe attack the next time. The severity is usually related to extra tension and strain and it is really very important to remain as calm as possible. Easier said than done, I know, particularly when you're in great pain.

Migraine can severely disrupt people's lives – from the disruption an attack can cause while at its peak, to the disruption that just worrying about a possible attack can bring with it. It's been known to lead to divorce when a partner shows little understanding. Planning holidays or travelling arrangements can become impossible. A fear of being taken ill in a strange place or not being able to find a darkened room to lie down in, can make a sufferer frightened to venture too far afield, either on holiday or to a social function. Or as one sixty-nine-year-old sufferer told me, 'My migraines became so bad that I was too frightened to go out, go anywhere, and much too frightened to drive. My life was hardly worth living.' And another, at just twenty years old, was driven to thoughts of suicide because migraine was controlling her life to such an extent that she felt lonely and isolated. Her young life, too, seemed hardly worth living.

WHAT CAUSES MIGRAINE?

Migraine (pronounced *me-graine* or *my-graine* – take your pick) causes such misery for so many people that I'm always being asked, 'What makes it more than "just a headache"?'

Well, for a start, the pain is usually one-sided and at the front of the head. It can occur on either side of the head and just because a sufferer has pain, say, on the left side, it doesn't necessarily follow that future attacks will always involve that particular side. In the 'common' type (now called migraine without aura) there are other symptoms such as loss of appetite, nausea or vomiting and concentration becomes extremely difficult. Sufferers have compared migraine to a storm that you know is gathering but there's nothing you can do about it. All you can do is let it take its course until it's blown itself out. Others have told me that the pain is so overwhelming they bang their head against a wall just to inflict another pain to distract them from the migraine's intense pain.

A few sufferers will have the 'classic' type of migraine (now called migraine with aura) preceded twenty to thirty minutes before the headache itself by warning symptoms – called an aura – which may include flashing lights before the eyes, shimmering or double vision, slurred speech, numbness and giddiness. Some figures suggest that only between about one in five and one in ten sufferers will have this type of migraine. In between attacks, sufferers will find themselves symptom-free.

It may seem strange, but although migraine really is a common problem, the *cause* of it isn't entirely understood. There is sometimes disagreement in the medical profession as to whether the cause is an abnormality in the way the brain controls the arteries in the body (opening them as well as closing them down) or an abnormality of the arteries themselves. The arteries particularly affected being the ones to the brain.

This is not to say that these blood vessels in the head are not a key source of the pain but rather to emphasise that changes in their diameter and/or the blood flow through them are not likely to play a causal role. Instead they represent one early step in the progression up to the full-blown attack, the real cause having started in the brain itself.

The key event believed to initiate a migraine attack is an inappropriate increase and/or fluctuation in the activity of specific nerves – called monoaminergic neurones – in response to a number of 'trigger factors'. Both the body's sympathetic nerves (part of our 'automatic' nervous system) and the lower part of our brain utilise a chemical called, for short, 5-HT. Between them, and with the involvement of the stress chemical noradrenaline, they control – via an even more complex chemical mechanism – the blood flow changes in the blood vessels both inside and outside the skull.

More significantly, the release of 5-HT from the nerves surrounding these blood vessels initiates and sustains an inflammatory process within the blood vessel wall – similar to that which could be caused by a germ invasion, for example.

The inflammation, as is usual, causes pain – and this pain is made worse by the release of what the researchers call substance P, a chemical released by the local tissues which 'enables' or enhances the pain message to be carried to the brain. It adds insult to injury and makes the pain and distress of a migraine attack into the scourge that it is.

You can see now just how complex the whole process is. Just to emphasise it, I should tell you that the key event that triggers the migraine also activates, in particular, the pain receptors – pain points if you like – on the sensation nerves of the face and scalp. It also provokes the local release of substances – as well as substance P – which allow those pain sensations and the vascular changes, characteristic of migraine, to be enhanced.

The associated nausea and/or vomiting is perhaps triggered by a release of 5-HT within the 'vomiting centre' in the brain. Alternatively, it could result from an increase in the sensations received from the Vagus nerve from the stomach, as a result of the release of 5-HT mobilised locally within the stomach and intestines.

Conclusion – the case for 5-HT being an important mediator in the study of migraine has strengthened in recent years. This is largely due to an increasing awareness, on the part of the researchers, of the effects on the workings of the body of the activation of many 5-HT receptor sites – places on the nerves and within the tissues where 5-HT can spark off the changes which result in a migraine.

But symptoms are probably due to a sudden constriction in some of the blood vessels in the brain. The headache comes on as these vessels then expand and the blood surges through this very sensitive organ, leading to the characteristic throbbing headache. Many experts believe that this constriction and dilation of the blood vessels is brought about by changing levels of certain chemicals circulating in the body, such as adrenaline – also released during stress – and prostaglandins. Adrenaline tenses the muscles, the heart and its blood vessels to prepare us for 'fight or flight'. Prostaglandins sensitise the nerve endings to make us more alert. In susceptible people, they will 'overdo' it and cause the above symptoms. Studies also suggest that there may be a slight difference – perhaps inherited – in the biochemical make-up of migraine sufferers which makes them more susceptible.

The trigger for an attack can be emotional or physical and common ones include anxiety, stress, excitement, depression, changes in weather or routine, bending for long periods (such as when gardening), hot baths, loud noises and flashing or bright light, including that from a VDU screen (glare filters are now available which many people find helpful). Alcohol, especially red wine, is one of the worst culprits, and certain foods, for example, chocolate, cheese, fried foods, citrus fruit, onions, tea, coffee, wheat flour, pork and seafood, are other common triggers.

Irregular meals, dieting or a long lie-in can provoke a migraine and some people also believe that close, thundery weather can cause them to have an attack. Or a change in the weather, say from a heavy shower of rain to sudden bright sunshine.

I have to advise you, though, that you shouldn't diagnose your own headache and label it migraine. The purpose of this book is not to diagnose it either. I merely seek to help migraine sufferers understand the problem in order to cope with it more easily. Your doctor is the only person who should decide what type of headache you're suffering from.

Headaches are an extremely common complaint, afflicting one person in three at least once a year, though some people do tend to suffer more than others. In fact, although we tend to use the word headache to describe any pain in the head, there are probably more than one hundred different types and they vary in intensity and location. Some develop gradually and clear up after an hour or two or a walk in the fresh air. Others can be extremely severe and can last more than twenty-four hours. Three of the commonest types of headache are migraine, of course, tension headache (sometimes known as muscle contraction headache) and sinus headache.

In a tension headache, the whole head throbs and feels as though there's a weight on top of it or a tight band around it. The pain is usually dull and persistent, originating in the muscles of the scalp. The tension headache is the most common symptom presented to a general practitioner and no one knows the cause, or why some people get a headache when they are emotionally upset and others don't.

A headache can also be brought on by other factors – drinking too much alcohol, anxiety or being in an overheated room or smoky atmosphere, or not having enough sleep. An illness such as 'flu or a cold can cause a headache. It may be the result of muscle strain in your neck, especially if the pain comes on after you have been reading or doing close work like sewing. Close work can also cause other types of facial-muscle strain – commonly thought of as eye-strain, which it isn't really. This can in turn lead to a headache. You can become tense from concentrating for too long or from sitting in an awkward position.

Another fairly common type is a sinus headache. In this type, pain tends to be dull and aching and stems from inflammation of the mucus membranes around the nose. These headaches can follow on from a head cold. Nasal congestion and catarrh – nasal discharge, or phlegm in the throat – are usually present for a few days during and after many infections of the nose and sinuses, especially the common cold. The combination is a harmless but annoying problem that can be stubborn to shift and can also result in deafness if it builds up in the eustachian tubes (the tubes on either side at the back of the nose and throat) which lead to the ears.

If your symptoms become more severe and the sinuses are infected, the condition is then called sinusitis. Anyone who has ever suffered from this will remember all too well the typical throbbing headache which is made worse by bending over or blowing the nose. It's estimated that one in two hundred colds leads to sinusitis.

The bones of the cheeks, forehead and back of the nose contain a hidden network of small caverns and channels – the sinuses – which help to make the bones lighter and give resonance to our voice. The mucus-secreting membrane that lines the nose continues on to form an inter-connecting lining for all the sinuses. Normally there is free movement and circulation of air into and from the nose and sinuses. Likewise, mucus can drain from the sinuses. When germs or particles of dirt are inhaled, they lodge in the mucus; minute, moving 'hairs' called cilia then waft them to the back of the nose where they are harmlessly swallowed (the stomach's secretions are highly acidic and instantly destroy most germs) or are blown out on to a handkerchief.

However, if the lining membrane of the sinuses becomes inflamed – which is quite common after a heavy cold – more mucus than usual is produced, the cilia cease to function properly, infected secretions build up, the tiny drainage holes may become blocked and acute sinusitis results. The pain can be similar to that caused by toothache and the affected sinus – along the cheekbone below the eye, or just above the eyebrow, for example – may be tender to the touch. The sufferer will probably feel generally unwell and have a nasty headache and a blocked nose.

An acute attack of sinusitis can usually be successfully treated by rest, painkillers and steam inhalations three times a day to relieve the congestion and help the sinuses to drain. For a severe attack antibiotics may be prescribed.

For most minor headaches, it's worth trying the following self-help measures. Take the recommended dose of a mild painkiller such as aspirin or paracetamol. For the best results, take the painkiller as soon as you feel the headache coming on. Drink plenty of water or other non-alcoholic, clear drinks. Rest in a quiet, darkened room may also be soothing and a warm bath will sometimes relieve tension.

Fortunately, most headaches are not a sign of a serious disease, but if your headache is particularly severe; if it's accompanied by misty or blurred vision, nausea or vomiting; if there's no satisfactory explanation for a headache that is continuous or getting worse after three days, or comes back several times in the course of a week; if it doesn't improve after taking a painkiller; or if you have injured your head during the past few days, you should consult your doctor for advice, and hopefully reassurance that there is nothing seriously wrong.

But when someone has worrying headaches, especially at first, the question at the forefront of their mind – and a frequent question to me – will usually be, 'Is this the start of a brain tumour?' Fortunately, the vast majority of headaches will be just that – headaches. And from what my readers tell me about the consultation they have had with their doctor, it is clear that he has excluded this usually remote possibility by his questions and examination. Your doctor will want to know various details about your headaches, such as when you had your first one of this nature; how often you have had one like this, and how long it's likely to last. He or she will also want to know whether or not the pain is on one side of your head, whether it moves around, what the pain is like and if you feel that there is something that may be triggering these attacks. He will also examine your eyes, ask you to 'follow his finger', and check your eye reflexes to light and distance vision.

By these means he is able to separate the symptom

– a headache – into its likely category and so provide further advice or treatment. Should he be at all concerned following the consultation, then he will request further investigations or a second opinion.

1: TYPES OF MIGRAINE

There are two common types of migraine: migraine with aura and the more frequent migraine without aura. The pain of the headache, which is described as the worst type of headache in the world, is equally intense whether it's with or without aura. Treatment either by conventional means or 'alternative' is the same, as are the self-help measures taken in order to cope. And although symptoms may vary slightly in each type, it's true to say that in between migraines sufferers do not have any symptoms, and that after some people have had several attacks of either kind of migraine, they can easily sense when another attack is imminent.

This kind of 'sixth sense', if you like, is actually referred to as 'premonitory symptoms'. These symptoms can surface in the day or two preceding the attack. Some people feel extremely well before a migraine and there can be mood changes, you feel either on a great high or a great low. Unexplained tiredness is another sign, as is feeling very fidgety, or craving a certain food, or being unable to stop yawning all the time, even being very talkative.

These premonitory symptoms can be helpful if a sufferer has discovered that taking medication at one of these first 'inklings' can prevent the full-scale migraine from developing, or may even prevent it altogether.

MIGRAINE WITH AURA

At the beginning of a migraine attack, sufferers experience what is called an 'aura', as I've mentioned earlier.

True to form, just as migraine itself varies in intensity and frequency from sufferer to sufferer, so can an aura. It can manifest itself as visual disturbances, such as flashing lights before the eyes; a tingling sensation in the fingers or up the arm; or a numbness in the arm spreading to the face. Some people find that speaking becomes difficult, others that they cannot see part of their usual field of vision, sometimes for as long as half an hour.

Auras can be frightening, especially when experienced for the first time, so it's helpful to understand what causes them and what is happening to your body at that time. The Migraine Trust quite rightly points out that symptoms such as pins and needles or numbness in the hand or arm can be quite unsettling in people with heart or circulatory disorders, as they can easily misinterpret the symptoms. For example, many people with chronic heart disease will experience discomfort or pain in their left hand or arm. The discomfort that can come with numbness may, to them, cause disquiet at best. They may fear that the heart pain of angina that they have suffered on a previous occasion may be about to return.

Likewise, numbness and pins and needles is a symptom often suffered by someone with vascular (circulation) problems in their limbs – usually in the legs. Having a migrainous cause, on top of their continuing circulatory problems, may turn an otherwise optimistic individual into an introspective worrier – and understandably so.

It's likely that the aura is brought on by the constriction in the blood vessels to the brain that occurs in the early stage of a migraine. The resulting restriction in the blood supply is probably the reason for the symptoms noted. Doctors call this reduction in blood supply to the tissues 'Ischaemia', and blood flow studies have shown reduced and increased flow respectively during the two stages of migraine.

Once the aura appears, a headache usually follows within an hour or so, as Lesley, a thirty-year-old housewife, now knows all too well. And her first aura is something she'll never forget nor the feelings of panic that went with it.

I was nineteen at the time and working as a temporary secretary during the college holidays. I'd heard of migraine but never really thought much about it and certainly didn't fully understand what the symptoms included. I just thought it was a bit of a bad headache, that people seemed to exaggerate about. People I worked with always seemed to be ringing in to take a day off sick because of a migraine.

To this day I can remember how frightened I was that afternoon. As I typed, I clearly remember the fingers of my left hand felt full of pins and needles. I thought initially that I'd been leaning on my wrist without realising and that my hand had gone to sleep. But then my hand went numb and this numbness spread slowly and surely up my arm.

At this stage my imagination ran riot. I thought I must be having a heart attack and when I tried to feel my heart beating with my right hand – I couldn't find it! I know it sounds ridiculous now but, believe me, I was convinced I was dying, in fact, that I was already dead! I was too frightened to tell anyone else in the office, because I knew I was being ridiculous and that they would think I was crazy. I just couldn't understand what was happening to me. I felt really peculiar, as if I wasn't quite there.

During the next hour or so Lesley sat still and quiet trying to calm down. To her relief the tingling sensations and numbness began to subside. But she wasn't prepared for what happened next.

That was when the most almighty headache I'd ever experienced began to take hold. So much for thinking people

exaggerate about migraine. It was so painful that even looking at the sheet of paper in my typewriter hurt my eyes. The
words I typed seemed to be trying to merge into each other.

I felt as if there was a tight metal band around my head
and someone was standing behind me tightening it,
although most of the pain was on the left side of my head.
My head was throbbing and at the same time I began to feel
like throwing up. The fluorescent lights in the room made
me feel even more uncomfortable. I couldn't bear to look
up at them, all I could do was screw my eyes up and look
down at my desk. After about an hour of suffering like this
I just had to get up and go home to bed. I instinctively
wanted to lie down somewhere dark and quiet.

MIGRAINE WITHOUT AURA

A migraine headache usually develops gradually while
building up in its intensity. Most sufferers find that the
pain tends to be on one side of the head only and often
describe it as pulsating, throbbing, pounding or even
hammering. Very often, for many sufferers, the
headache develops as they wake up in the morning –
goodness knows why. According to the Migraine Trust,
recent studies have suggested that migrainous subjects
are habitually likely to seek out and experience high levels of information input – that is, by personality they are
people who seek knowledge, interest, activity and are
less content just to sit.

The nature of this information – for example, verbal,
spatial, auditory or visual – may determine which part
and which side of the brain is optimally involved in the
process at any one time. Such individuals, due to waken
with migraine, have been found, during the latter part of
their sleep, to develop a surge of noradrenaline in their
plasma at a time when normally such levels are falling.
Eventually they waken from a period of REM

– Rapid Eye Movement activity – when a researcher can observe their eyes moving under their lids as they reach the lighter, second phase of sleep. (These sleep phases are also defined by the electrical impulses given off by the brain. They can be measured by an instrument called an EEG – an Electro EncephaloGram. It is during phase two sleep that we dream.)

It has been suggested that the developments associated with mounting vascular disturbance in the relevant part of the brain may reflect a faltering of the brain's capacity to assimilate an excessive amount of information, either on account of that excess or else because of its challenge in emotional terms – the 'worry' about how we will be able to cope with it.

Possibly a migraine which erupts during wakefulness is also brought on if such REM periods, which occur naturally every ninety minutes or so throughout the night, are not stable enough to be satisfying, so we have too many even lighter periods of sleep – very close to wakefulness – and thus get a migraine.

But I'm not convinced by these suggestions. We don't really know is my view.

Many sufferers have told me that they tend to lose interest in eating during a migraine attack, which is understandable if the headache is accompanied by the unpleasant sensation of nausea. But it's also referred to medically as anorexia or loss of appetite. There is evidence also that the stomach 'closes down' as an attack begins. Nevertheless, it does help to try to eat small quantities of food during an attack. Many sufferers have told me that after a migraine they feel the lack of food – sometimes for as long as twenty-four hours – makes them feel even worse, often weak and dehydrated. If you can, try to eat something containing carbohydrate. This is because it is bland to the digestive system and is slowly turned into simple sugars as part of the digestive process. This provides the body with a ready supply of energy 'fuel' that will help it to overcome the symptoms.

Some people vomit frequently during an attack, others find that once they vomit the migraine has reached its peak and is likely to be drawing to a close. I'm often asked whether you can have migraine without having nausea and vomiting. The answer is, yes. These two unpleasant symptoms may not necessarily accompany an attack.

Resting in a darkened room is helpful for most people, probably because a migraine involves a sensitivity to brightness and light, called photophobia. People who suffer from migraine can also dislike bright lights in between attacks and can find lights provoke a migraine.

Scott, a sixty-four-year-old retired plumber and a migraine sufferer for forty years, finds bright natural light as well as artificial light can trigger a migraine attack. He also is extremely photophobic once an attack has begun.

When I have a migraine I either have to wear dark glasses or rest in a dark room. Glare of all kinds can be irritating beyond belief. I can't even try to look at light, I find it almost blinding.

But it's not only when I have an attack. In winter I find that when I wake up in the morning and my wife turns on the light I have to cover my eyes because if I don't that sudden bright light could give me a migraine. In the summer, I have to be careful not to look out of the bedroom window first thing in the morning if it's bright and sunny. If I did my vision would go – my eyesight becomes blurred and I know I'm going to develop a headache within about ten minutes.

Dazzling reflected light is another trigger. I have to be careful to avoid looking at light reflected off other cars on a sunny day, or if there has been a shower of rain and then the sun comes out I immediately put on dark glasses to cut down on the glare.

If I watch television for too long – say, if I decide to watch an evening of television because I have nothing else to do, or I want to relax, I can only watch it for about three hours. If I watch any more I know I'll get a migraine. Watching television when the screen is too bright or the picture has a very slight flicker triggers an attack, too.

And I absolutely hate fluorescent lights and disco lights. I can't stay for very long in any place with fluorescent lights, for example department stores. The effect is even worse when a store has low ceilings as well. My wife and I always seem to be invited to weddings or other functions where there's a disco. I really don't like to go – my wife accuses me of being anti-social. But I cannot bear coloured, flashing disco lights or those strange strobe lights that some disk jockeys seem to enjoy using. They make my life a misery.

Dislike of light is not the only additional aspect of a migraine attack. People can experience diarrhoea or constipation. They can be more sensitive to noise or smells, or their hearing seems to become much more keen. The slightest noise, or trying to sleep while someone is watching the television downstairs, for instance, can become extremely irritating. Many sufferers find that it can be difficult to think and concentration becomes impossible. This is made even worse when you are trying to struggle on at work until you can leave for home, painkillers and bed.

But the trouble doesn't stop for many people once the migraine attack has drawn to a close. Once a migraine is over you can feel worn out, and one sufferer told me that her brain feels 'spongy' for a couple of days afterwards. Others find that they don't feel 100 per cent but are so relieved to be able to go out again and carry on their normal routine that they quickly overdo things and trigger off another attack.

CLUSTER HEADACHES

Cluster headaches can also be called migrainous neuralgia. This type of headache is not uncommon and very unpleasant as the attacks occur together in clusters or runs which can last for weeks or months at a time with periods of relief in between. Men – usually in the thirty- to forty-year age group – are more likely to develop this rare type of migraine than women. Sufferers often wake up in the early morning with a headache, which has caused these attacks sometimes to be referred to as 'alarm clock headaches'.

The pain often centres in the eye, the face or the neck and may last for twenty to sixty minutes, though the variation from one sufferer to another is quite large. The skin may flush, the eyes weep, the nose may become congested and blood vessels may be enlarged on the whites of the eyes.

HEMIPLEGIC MIGRAINE

Sometimes the aura and associated symptoms preceding or accompanying the migraine attack may be so marked that the one-sided neurological signs of numbness, pins and needles and even temporary paralysis may resemble the signs and symptoms associated with a stroke – or hemiplegia. Hence the name. Fortunately this type of migraine should get better within hours and the paralysis is not as marked as that which occurs with a stroke.

BASILAR MIGRAINE

This is a form of classical migraine in which the aura or prodromal symptoms – any symptoms which arise before the full-blown attack – originate from the arteries in the neck and the base of the skull. The pain is commonly felt right at the back of the head – known as the Occiput. The symptoms can be frightening to say the least, including the loss of control over one's walking ability, which doctors call ataxia, pins and needles and numbness on both sides of the body, not just one. There can also be dizziness, double vision, impaired speech and a temporary loss of consciousness. It mainly affects young adults. Understandably, both the sufferer and any onlookers are worried out of their skins.

OPTHALMOPLEGIC MIGRAINE

Another one of the frighteners. This causes a temporary paralysis of the nerves which move the eyeball within its socket. This can lead to drooping eyelids, a dilated pupil, double vision and an inability to move the eyes in some or all directions. A sufferer will usually prefer to keep their eyes closed. These symptoms can outlast the headache by many days so that the doctors, even the specialists and all connected, are deeply concerned that the severity of the symptoms and signs are such that a definite defect within the skull, leading to longer-lasting defects – a blood-vessel blowout, for example – is the cause. Occasionally these gruesome symptoms will be made even worse by a patch or patches of blindness – called a scotoma. What's more, these attacks can re-occur, though when they do all concerned will be more confident of the diagnosis, which is something to be grateful for at least.

INFREQUENT MIGRAINES

Some sufferers may be fortunate in that they do not have attacks that often – sometimes as infrequently as once a year or less. It really does differ from person to person, just as the length of an attack varies from several hours to several days. The saying 'There's an exception to every rule' really does apply to migraine, but goodness knows why this is so.

Mark, a thirty-nine-year-old local government officer, has experienced only a few migraine attacks in the last five years – they are not that frequent but two of them were severe and unpleasant enough for him to dread another developing. He's found that the attacks arrived totally unexpectedly. He had no aura, no premonitory symptoms and certainly cannot trace any trigger factors.

Two attacks stick in his memory particularly – one on a hot summer's day.

The initial sign that something was wrong was when I felt that my body was in no way connected to my legs. It was a very hot day and I was walking across a large open area of playing fields. I can even remember looking down at my legs and being surprised that they were taking me along, I felt as if I was floating. Within minutes I had an excruciating throbbing pain in the right part of my skull. It was as if my head had enlarged so that if I put my hand up to touch my forehead it would be about an inch further out than it should have been.

My only solace was to cup my forehead with my hand. Somehow I managed to drive home very carefully and immediately undressed and got into bed. I woke up five or six hours later as if the whole incident had never happened. It was as if there had been total electrical shut down in my brain.

More recently, while driving, Mark developed such a violent headache accompanied with such severe nausea that he had to stop immediately and rush to the side of the road to be sick.

The headache started off as a run-of-the-mill type and then it became turbo-charged and grew in strength. I was just driving along, at around midday, when my headache started. This time I was certain that it was going into migraine mode and within half an hour it had reached its peak. I felt so terrible I had to stop the car at a bus stop and get out so that I could vomit.

It was so embarrassing to be seen retching and vomiting into a bush at the side of the road. Yet in some ways at the time I couldn't have cared less because of the relief it was giving me. When I've had a migraine I find that either vomiting or opening my bowels eases the problem. Somehow that all seems to relieve the pressure which is almost inflating my body and adding to the sensation that my forehead is being pushed forward from its normal position. But I hadn't vomited in public since I was a child – I loathe the thought of it happening to me again.

Since I have now experienced a few attacks I do fear the arrival of an attack so much that if I have the slightest headache I immediately take painkillers and that seems to stop anything further developing.

2: TRIGGER FACTORS

Just as the duration and intensity of a migraine attack can vary between individuals, so do trigger factors. Mention migraine and people automatically jump to the assumption that the triggers are just chocolate and red wine. But many sufferers can eat chocolate, even drink red wine – it's really a question of detective work if you want to be able to pinpoint the trigger factor in your case. Being able to avoid triggers can reduce the frequency and severity of attacks, especially if avoidance is carried out while you're also taking medication. So many people try a prescription medicine from their GP then promptly forget that it's still worth being strict about trigger factors. You shouldn't rely just on your medication to control migraines.

These are commonly accepted examples of trigger factors, which you can start off by looking out for:

food
alcohol
changes in the weather
bright or flickering lights
hormones – menstruation or the menopause
smells – perfume, for example
psychological factors – stress, worry, mental
    fatigue, etc
going on a diet
skipped meals
too much or too little sleep
taking a very hot bath
high blood pressure
a change in routine – such as getting up very early

physical or mental fatigue
relaxation after stress
holidays and weekends

Don't be surprised if you find more than one trigger factor, or a definite combination. For example, one sufferer discovered he could sometimes drink a glass of red wine without any ill-effect, but at other times it triggered a migraine. He eventually found that if he had a glass of red wine on a Friday evening after a particularly busy week, as well as not having eaten much that day, he'd develop a migraine the following morning.

MIGRAINE AND FOOD

It has been well established that migraine can be triggered by certain foods – although some experts believe that only one in ten migraine sufferers find that their attacks are indeed set off by it. So it's important to understand that food isn't the main cause of migraine, though in some people it very often triggers attacks.

Food known to trigger migraines includes chocolate, alcohol (particularly red wine), cheese, citrus fruits, nuts, meats, dairy products, coffee and tea, monosodium glutamate, shellfish and fried foods. Of course, other foods can trigger migraine attacks in individuals – some sufferers have even traced their sensitivity down to the humble onion family, pork, or sharp unripe green apples. Cutting out wheat-containing products from the diet has helped other sufferers. As you can see, it really is a matter of trial and error as what can affect one person may not cause migraine in another. For some sufferers, food may not even play a part in their migraines at all.

Chocolate and cheese, red wine or sherry – all of

which contain a lot of tyramine (or similar chemicals in the case of chocolate) – are famous migraine triggers. These chemicals are similar to adrenaline, which is known to set off the illness. However one report in the Lancet in the late 1980s suggested that a chemical called phenolic flavanoids (which gives red wine its colour) could be responsible. This leaks from grape skins and pips during the making. White wine isn't affected as much because the skins and pips are separated from the juice early on.

For the scientifically minded, these flavanoids inhibit the body's enzyme that detoxifies a particular group of chemicals and phenols in the intestine, chemicals which we could well do without. A build-up of these can cause migraine/headache symptoms.

Apparently, in older wines – mature claret, for example – flavanoids form chains making them into bigger molecules, that is, larger chemical particles which are not therefore absorbed. This is likely to be the reason why those fortunate enough to afford the better wines do claim that a surfeit does not cause the other characteristic symptoms of the 'morning after' – symptoms totally unrelated to migraine, though quite unpleasant nevertheless (I believe!). Some sufferers do confirm that cheap red wine gives them a migraine while expensive wines do not.

So, as you can see, chemicals found within food can trigger migraine, and it's not just the chemicals in cheese, chocolate or wine. Some people find that they develop a migraine after eating a Chinese meal or cured meats, for example, or a hot dog. A food additive such as monosodium glutamate is frequently used as a flavour enhancer in Chinese cooking and this can be a migraine trigger. The additive is found in many ready-made sauces as well as stock cubes. So it's worth spending a few moments in the supermarket checking a product's list of ingredients if you feel monosodium glutamate affects you. In cured meats (this category includes bacon, ham and salami) nitrites may have been added to the salt that's used in the curing process. Nitrites are chemicals known as vasodilators which widen blood vessels.

Surprisingly, perhaps, ice-cream too can give some people a migraine. This is to do with temperature rather than contents: the cold feeling on the roof of the mouth can produce a referred pain – a pain felt in another part of the nerves' 'territory' although it's not really coming from there – and so cause a headache.

While some people find, to their disappointment, that food has nothing to do with provoking their migraines, other sufferers have been more fortunate and have been able to pinpoint quite accurately what foods need to be omitted from their diet.

Sian, a twenty-seven-year-old secretary, was so fed up with migraine that she decided to eliminate slowly all the foods that allegedly triggered it. She was one of the lucky ones – she was able to work out quite precisely which foods she had to avoid to prevent a migraine attack. For the past three years she has been able to enjoy life without migraines unless she lets her diet 'rules' slip slightly.

I'd been told by a doctor that I had a migraine-related allergy to alcohol, so I knew that had to be my starting point. When I was a student and would go to parties I would only have two or three drinks, perhaps lager, or Dubonnet and lemonade, a Martini or wine, and I would begin to feel so sick within about an hour. Or if I didn't feel sick then I would go to bed and dream that I was feeling nauseous and eventually wake to run to the bathroom where I wouldn't be able to stop vomiting. I'd usually have a headache the next morning, but the headache wasn't as bad to cope with as the vomiting.

My friends used to think it was a bit of a joke really and I used to get ever so fed up about it, especially as people used to imply that I was a bit neurotic or just a hypochondriac. I'd try not to drink when we all went out but you're made to feel a bit of a social outcast when you continually refuse a drink, even a glass of wine. At parties friends were always pressurising me to have a glass of wine, and then another. So often I used to end up with a migraine the next day just because I gave in to their demands. I didn't want to feel the odd one out all the time.

I'd read that pure spirits like vodka and gin are supposedly less likely to give you migraine than something such as red wine or brandy. I tried on several occasions just having a vodka or one gin and tonic and my headache was just as terrible the following morning. No matter what alcoholic drink I tried, the effect always seemed to be the same, although looking back I suppose red wine was the very worst culprit.

I remember one wedding I went to and our glasses were constantly filled with red wine. It may be hard to believe this but I had a headache that lasted a week after that. It was awful. I felt as if someone was squeezing the backs of my eyeballs until they were forced out of my head. Anyway, after that wedding I decided not to drink for a whole year, no matter what anyone said – and not even at Christmas. And I stuck to it. That's how determined I was.

Although her migraines did decrease by cutting out all alcohol from her diet they didn't stop altogether, and Sian was determined to track down what else might be triggering them.

I'd read that citrus fruits could trigger migraine and I used to drink freshly squeezed orange juice every day. So I cut that out as well as cutting out eating satsumas and tangerines. That definitely made a difference within a couple of weeks.

A friend told me that coffee and tea were supposed to be bad for migraine because of the caffeine content. And that even a cup, rather than a mug, of strong tea can contain a very high dose of caffeine. I'd only ever drunk very weak tea, and not that often, so cutting out that didn't make much difference. But at the time, we used to drink a lot of instant coffee at work, which I didn't particularly like but drank out of convenience whenever I fancied a break from work. I decided to try giving it up for a while and to switch to real coffee. Amazingly that made quite a difference. Even now I can't drink instant coffee but real ground coffee doesn't affect me at all. Cutting out chocolate made a difference, too, although I found that I could eat chocolate in moderation, and it was only when I had a combination of things, like chocolate, coffee and say a glass of wine, that it would trigger a migraine. Although I did notice after a while that if I had a bar of chocolate instead of a proper meal, say, because I was rushing around the shops in my lunch hour and hadn't had time to get a sandwich, it could mean I would get a migraine.

It's likely that the caffeine in tea and coffee, being a stimulant, excites both the central nervous system as well as the body's production of its stress hormones – including adrenaline and up to twenty others called catechol amines. It's probably these that are able to trigger a migraine in the susceptible. Many sufferers tend to forget, to their disadvantage, about the caffeine in their tea or coffee when they are trying to eliminate triggers from their diet.

And what Sian perhaps didn't know is that chocolate contains theobromine, another stimulant, which is very similar to caffeine both in its composition as well as the effects it has upon our bodily functions. That's why the chocolate bar was triggering a migraine. She continued:

I also discovered that I could eat cheese, particularly types like fromage frais or a not very ripe Brie, and other soft cheeses, yet a hard cheese like a very mature Cheddar would give me a headache. My doctor told me that was because different cheeses have different amounts of tyramine. He explained that tyramine is thought to dilate blood vessels so resulting in a migraine attack.

Yet the biggest culprit of all, apart from alcohol, instant coffee and orange juice, was yoghurt. Typically I absolutely love the stuff, but just one pot of strawberry yoghurt would give me the most violent migraine the following day. It's funny to think that something so innocent-looking and supposedly with such a healthy image should make me feel so ill!

I have to be honest and say that I was disheartened to find that things I particularly like, like red wine and yoghurt, gave me migraine (and still could), but on the other hand I was so pleased to be able to track down these trigger factors and doing without them is much easier than putting up with migraine.

By the end of that year I really could keep my migraines under control. I was even able to have the odd glass of white wine now and again and get away with it. From then on I found that I would get a migraine right out of the blue – or so it seemed. Yet when I sat down and thought about it, I realised that most of the time they occurred when I'd been a bit sloppy about watching what I had been eating. I still found that occasionally I would have a migraine if I had been quite worried about something. But, for instance, I might have had a glass of orange juice one day, then a bar of chocolate the next, followed by an instant coffee at a friend's house because I hadn't felt like making a fuss and saying I couldn't really drink instant coffee. The memories of my student days when I was sometimes labelled a bit neurotic still haunt me and I hardly ever let on to anyone that I get migraines. It's ridiculous really that I still prefer to suffer the consequences of eating or drinking a trigger factor rather than make a fuss in front of other people, but that's the way it is. And I know a lot of other migraine sufferers feel the same way. Sometimes I feel we're our own worst enemies!

I'd only have a few seemingly trivial lapses but the cumulative effect produced a migraine. These days I'm beginning to be much more careful and, for instance, rather than say instant coffee gives me a headache when I'm offered it, I'll just refuse and say I'd rather have a glass of water or a cup of tea. It's easier that way because I know some people don't really sympathise, especially if they've never had a migraine.

While we're talking about food and migraine, I think it's worth pointing out here that some specialists now believe that a reduced blood sugar level is a more common trigger than chocolate, cheese, alcohol and the like, particularly in the cases of childhood migraines and menstrual migraines. That's why skipping meals, not eating enough in a day or dieting can trigger attacks.

I believe that we shall hear a lot more about the effects of low blood sugar – hypoglycaemia – before too long, even though there are other specialists who consider that food allergy far out-strips hypoglycaemia as a trigger. I now have an open mind on both issues.

In America and on the continent they have long believed in 'physiological' hypoglycaemia as a cause of many common symptoms – that during those times when hypoglycaemia is likely to occur (for example in the late morning and after no breakfast, or an inadequate one), migraine, dizziness, panic attacks including nausea, not to mention feelings of anxiety or apprehension could be the result.

But doctors in the UK – me included – have been sceptical. We do not consider that the scientific evidence is strong enough for this to be so. The normal concentration of sugar – glucose – in the blood does vary quite widely throughout the day, but still remains within normal limits in all healthy people. So the question we have to ask ourselves is why it is that not everyone experiences the symptoms mentioned above since we all have periods when our blood sugar concentration is equally low. And I don't know the answer to that one.

But if someone finds that they don't get a migraine and other symptoms if they eat regular meals and so keep their blood sugar levels from hitting the floor, then what have we got to lose by accepting the theory? As long as it doesn't stop us looking for others that could be more specific.

So if you find that a low blood sugar level affects the frequency of your migraines, you should try to eat regularly – don't go more than three hours without eating something. It's always handy to keep a snack in your handbag, or briefcase, as a standby to save you being caught out. If you know you are likely to be a few hours without food – for example, if you are going out for the evening – then try to make sure that you eat something before you go. Even if you are going to a friend's house for dinner, you needn't spoil your appetite. Just have a snack so that you don't have to worry about what time food is going to be served.

If you are one of those people who just cannot face food first thing in the morning, and have never eaten breakfast, do try to eat and drink something during the morning. Some sufferers find that only eating a sandwich for lunch isn't enough to avert a migraine attack. If you think this is the case, then always try to have a cooked lunch no matter how small – you don't have to have three courses!

MIGRAINE AND STRESS

Stress is a common trigger factor in attacks of migraine. Stress to one person may not be stress to another. As many sufferers have told me, sometimes they're not even aware they're under stress until the migraine strikes. One sufferer, a mother of two, always has a migraine during the first couple of days of a holiday.

She couldn't understand why this should be so during a 'relaxing' time. But when she took into account the run-up to the holiday, the preparation – not least the family washing, ironing and packing – and her children's over-excitement, she realised she'd been pretty stressed without even noticing it.

Of course, it's not always possible to remove stress factors from your life as it affects us all every day, not just before we go on holiday. And from all the calls I receive on the *Jimmy Young Show*, as well as letters I'm sent regularly, I've reached the conclusion that recognising that we're stressed, why we should be so and then acting to solve the problem, isn't easy for anyone. It can be hard for many people just to admit that they feel stressed – so often they feel it's viewed as a sign of weakness, or of not being able to do their job properly, or a confession that they are in fact feeling very lonely.

However, stress isn't always a bad thing. Positive stress, or pressure, is needed for us to work well and to drive us to get the most out of life. That rush of adrenaline everyone will recognise stimulates and motivates. For many people, having no rush of adrenaline makes their lives feel boring, mundane and can even make lethargy and depression more likely.

Your personality and just the way you're made can decide how much stress you can take – but that doesn't mean to say that migraine sufferers can't tolerate pressure or are made in a different way to everybody else.

I'm sure many readers have heard of the fight or flight response of cavemen. Our bodies have an automatic response to fear or pleasure, releasing the hormones adrenaline and noradrenaline. These cause the heart rate to increase as well as providing instant energy by causing sugars and fats to be let into the blood. As cavemen we would stay and fight the man or animal causing us stress, or we would run away. Not very practical reactions these days! So because we can't 'flee' or 'fight', the body's adrenaline is bottled up instead. And, as I've mentioned, this stress does seem to be a common trigger for migraine sufferers.

For many, a period of stress is often inevitably followed by a migraine – usually when they are beginning to unwind. Very often people who have high-powered jobs, or jobs that they find particularly stressful, have a regular weekend migraine. That is, come Friday evening, when the pressures of the week are starting to fade and the person is beginning to relax, a migraine attack will creep up. If not on Friday night, certainly for many people it will be there once they wake on Saturday morning.

It's unusual for a migraine sufferer not to be able to take a driving test, for instance, or an important examination. Yet once the period of stress is over they are quite likely to have an attack. Having said that, of course, there are exceptions to this rule and some sufferers will inevitably have a migraine when they least want one.

Katherine, a thirty-four-year-old journalist, found that whenever her job involved a stressful working trip, she coped while she had to, but once she came home and the pressure was off, she'd have a violent migraine headache.

I remember one trip was particularly bad. It was when I was working on a weekly women's magazine. The atmosphere on the magazine wasn't cosy and sweet as many people seemed to think it might be. Instead it was a very competitive environment and we all worked particularly hard, with constant tough deadlines to meet.

At this particular time, I had to go to Belfast for a week to do a series of different interviews and features. Of course, I was quite nervous about going to Northern Ireland –

I didn't even tell members of my family about it, because I didn't want them to worry, too.

While I was there I really enjoyed myself. The people were very friendly, although I was quite shocked by the poverty I saw and the aggressive murals painted on walls in both Catholic and Protestant areas. At one point the photographer and I got totally lost in West Belfast. It's almost impossible to find your way around even with a map because so many roads have street blocks or are cordoned off. It was pretty nerve-wracking, especially as it was in the dead of night and the photographer was as nervous as I was, which didn't help. Another day we had travelled outside Belfast and were stopped by an Army patrol while a helicopter hovered overhead. The soldiers searched our car, including all the photographer's equipment. They insisted on listening to my tape recorder. A woman soldier even searched through my hair to look for, as she said, anything a terrorist might be trying to hide! I have to admit that was pretty nerve-wracking, too. But I wasn't aware that I was that frightened, or stressed.

It was only when I came home that I realised just how much pressure I'd been under. Not only was it quite frightening to be in Northern Ireland but I was under pressure to do all the interviews well and make sure I came back to work with good stories. The day after my return I awoke with the most severe migraine headache I had ever had. I felt so nauseous I couldn't even get out of bed and in fact I had to stay there for two days before I felt well enough to move. So much for thinking of myself as an intrepid reporter!

3: MIGRAINE AND WOMEN

MIGRAINE AND HORMONES – PREMENSTRUAL SYNDROME

Premenstrual tension (PMT) is increasingly becoming known as premenstrual syndrome. The word 'syndrome' is more accurate, because there are so many different symptoms associated with the changes before a period, not just the well-documented feelings of tension.

Premenstrual syndrome is a complex set of many different symptoms, both physical and emotional, which occur in the two weeks before menstruation. Because of the wide range of these symptoms, from migraine to constipation, anxiety or just tiredness, many doctors in the past have not recognised PMS, and women have been put on tranquillisers inappropriately.

PMS is due to a hormonal imbalance which takes place regularly each month as the body adjusts itself in readiness for menstruation. Unlike men, whose hormone levels are constant, women's hormone levels change constantly throughout their reproductive lives. This could be the trigger factor for migraine and the reason why more women suffer than men.

PMS can start right from the first period, or when there's been a gap between periods, during the vast hormonal changes after pregnancy, following artificial changes in the hormonal balance with the pill, or sterilisation (although it shouldn't, scientifically) or if your periods have stopped due to an illness.

For many women one of the most distressing and frightening symptoms is loss of control over their feelings – otherwise gentle women have become violent towards their children and partners. Some, totally out of character, have even committed crimes while suffering, particularly shoplifting.

But many women find that migraine forms part of their premenstrual symptoms and that their migraines become worse just before a period, or they inevitably develop in the two days prior to the period. Most also develop migraines at other times as well – some women, for example, find migraines occur when they ovulate. It's been estimated by some experts that as many as two-thirds of female migraine sufferers believe that their menstrual cycle affects the incidence of their migraines. You can see how hormones must play a part in the condition when you consider that before puberty the ratio of boys to girls with migraine is equal, yet it becomes more common in girls once menstruation has commenced.

There is no 'cure' for PMS, but there is now a variety of possible treatments which either treat individual symptoms – sometimes diuretics, used temporarily, for the feelings of bloatedness associated with water retention – or which help reduce the hormonal imbalances that lead to all sorts of unpleasant symptoms (see page 66 for what your doctor may prescribe). Period time migraines often respond to treatment with the hormone progesterone, see page 66. You should try not to miss meals, and should avoid any other factor that you know triggers an attack. Eating well is important, too, as a healthy, regular, well-balanced diet with plenty of fresh fruit and vegetables can only be good for you – and keeps your blood sugar levels topped up.

If you feel your migraines are menstrually related then it really is a good idea to keep a diary (see page 91). By recording a note of your attacks you'll be able to tell whether or not your migraine does fall into a definite sequence.

Work carried out at the City of London Migraine Clinic has found that the link between migraine and menstruation becomes stronger in the years just before the menopause. It seems that for many women migraines were not linked to their periods in their younger years but from their mid to late thirties the attacks began to fall into a monthly pattern.

MIGRAINE AND THE PILL

I'm often asked whether migraine can be a side-effect of the pill? The contraceptive pill has been the subject of more research, publicity and controversy than probably any other medicine. This is partly because, unlike other medicines, it is taken by healthy women and not to cure or relieve symptoms, so any risk involved is less acceptable. However, many people choose to continue smoking in spite of the known, far greater risks and widely used medicines, such as aspirin, are also potentially far more harmful than the pill. Take an overdose of the pill and you will come to no lasting harm, whereas an overdose of aspirin could be fatal.

Although undoubtedly the pill is not suitable for all women, the ultra low-dose pills now available and the tri-phasic pills (the dosage in these is related to the natural ebb and flow of the woman's hormones) have helped reduce any risks and side-effects to a minimum. Studies done over the thirty years since the pill has been in use have also given doctors clearer and safer guidelines for prescribing it so that women at any particular risk can be singled out and an alternative method of contraception advised. For millions of women, however, the pill continues to be a simple, reversible and virtually 100 per cent effective method for which they are thankful.

There are two main types of pill: the most commonly used combined pill (which contains a combination of the two hormones oestrogen and progestogen) and the so-called 'mini-pill'. The latter is not, as some people believe, just a low-dose combined pill, but is altogether different as it contains only one hormone – progestogen – and acts in quite a different way to prevent conception. When taking the combined pill, the circulating hormones normally 'trick' the body into thinking it has already ovulated. The ovaries do not therefore receive their usual 'message' to release an egg – so, no egg, no pregnancy. The pill's other effects – upon the lining of the womb – prevent a pregnancy on those occasions when ovulation does occur.

The mini-pill may also prevent ovulation but its main effect is to alter the consistency of the mucus within the cervix (the entrance to the womb) making it thick and impenetrable to the sperm. It acts, in other words, as a kind of barrier method. For the mucus to maintain this impenetrable consistency, it is important to take this type of pill about the same time each day.

Until recently, when a woman reached the age of thirty-five, doctors would advise her against taking the 'combined' contraceptive pill. This was because of the much increased risk of a venous thrombosis (an unusual clot forming in a vein) associated with the previous higher dosed pills. An alternative sometimes suggested was the progestogen-only mini-pill, but because this can make the periods irregular, or stop them altogether, anxiety about possible pregnancy is often a problem. So the choices available to the older couple, if they wished to avoid pregnancy until the menopause, were limited. Now a new pill is available formulated for women over thirty. It contains only 20 micrograms of oestrogen – a third less than the usual

30 microgram pills. The combination with a new type of progestogen (desogestrel), carefully balanced, enables it to be just as effective as other pills. It is recommended for older women as their particular menstrual cycles are usually well regulated even by this low level of oestrogen, which also has health advantages. Studies show that desogestrel benefits the skin and also appears to have a favourable effect on some of the risk factors associated with heart disease and strokes. The smaller doses of oestrogen mean that some common side-effects of the usual pills – breast tenderness and nausea, for example – are less likely.

Unfortunately, the health risks of the pill have been more publicised than the health benefits and figures show that 91 per cent of women in the older age group think that the pill is unsafe for them. Actually, research has proved that it does protect against cancer of the womb and the ovaries, makes fibroids less likely, prevents vaginal dryness (and so can improve sex life), controls symptoms such as hot flushes in the years leading up to the menopause, and prevents osteoporosis – thinning of the bones. As a result of these findings, family planning experts now advise that as long as a woman is fit there is no reason why she should not enjoy these benefits until the age of forty-five or even until the menopause. The trend towards a healthier lifestyle – improved eating habits, regular exercise and no smoking – is now making more and more women suitable for the pill.

Full discussion with your doctor and health screening checks such as regular cervical smears and blood pressure checks are needed before deciding whether (and for how long) the pill is right for you. However, with the low-dose ones now available and the reassuring evidence of their safety, it certainly could be.

It's quite common for migraine to be associated with the pill and the condition can be aggravated by it – although for other women the pill can actually *prevent* migraine symptoms, rather than make them worse.

But if you develop migraine for the first time while you are taking the contraceptive pill, you should discuss it with your doctor, to establish whether it's advisable to carry on with this type of contraception. If you are already a migraine sufferer and your migraine becomes worse then you should definitely seek your doctor's advice, and without delay.

But on balance, most doctors will probably advise someone whose migraine is bad, or who experiences aura – a tingling or numbness in the limbs and/or visual disturbance – or whose migraine becomes worse when they take the pill, to use another method of contraception, and I agree with them.

MIGRAINE AND PREGNANCY

It's sometimes said that pregnancy can improve your migraines. About three-quarters of female migraine sufferers find that their headaches subside during pregnancy, and it's rare for migraine to develop for the first time in a women who's pregnant. This is likely to be due to the anti-inflammatory effect of the large doses of female hormones which are coursing around the body at these times. But that can't be the precise reason otherwise the oral contraceptive would *always* relieve migraine, and it doesn't.

And it seems to me that each woman's response is varied. Some women have found that their migraines have stopped during pregnancy and after childbirth, but others have been disappointed to find that although their migraines stopped during the nine months of pregnancy they returned about three months after giving birth.

And specialists have discovered that in pregnancy the sex hormone levels show profound changes. The oestrogen levels can sometimes reach one hundred times the normal, non-pregnant level, while progesterone levels decrease but rise again towards the end of pregnancy. However, they don't fluctuate up and down so rapidly or so much at these times and this may be why migraine improves during pregnancy.

Another possible protection against headache attacks might be the body's own natural painkillers – the morphine-like opioids. During pregnancy these substances, more specifically known as endorphins, can be several times higher than usual but, after delivery, rapidly decline and headaches recur.

During pregnancy, your doctor will advise you when he believes that medication is essential. On the general grounds that all unnecessary medicines should be avoided, especially in the early stages, seek his advice before taking anything.

MIGRAINE AND THE MENOPAUSE

The menopause, referred to as 'the change' or the 'change of life', comes about when the ovaries stop producing the female hormone oestrogen. The most common symptoms are hot flushes and night sweats. These can be accompanied by mood swings and sleeping problems and the vagina can become dry as secretions lessen, causing soreness. Headaches, too, can be a common symptom. Unfortunately, there is no guarantee that migraine is going to stop at the menopause, though it's true to say that it often does become less severe and even disappears for some sufferers. However one study of women suffering from migraine after the menopause showed that a quarter of them began suffering from the problem *after* the change of life.

Symptoms of the menopause can be relieved by hormone replacement therapy. I believe that HRT – supplementing the hormone oestrogen which women stop producing during the menopause – is one of the best medical breakthroughs of the past twenty years or so. In my opinion, the day will come when HRT will be compared favourably with other replacement medicines that are required when the body fails to produce its own – such as the thyroid hormone and even insulin, with its life-saving properties for the diabetic.

While only one in five women experiences excessive menopausal symptoms, like hot flushes and depression, at least another one or two in five will suffer less severe characteristics – emotional and social, as well as physical – which they don't necessarily relate to the menopause until they've tried HRT and discovered the difference in the way they feel. Of course, HRT will not necessarily overcome the apprehension felt at the passing of the years, but it does help a great number of women to feel more optimistic about the prospect, and to have confidence in themselves.

It's not just the symptoms of the menopause that will be relieved, either. An unacceptable proportion of women in later years develop osteoporosis – commonly known as brittle bones – and HRT can prevent this. Osteoporosis causes not only thinning of the bones, but also more distressing changes, like the spine bending to produce a hump at the top. This causes the woman to lose height, and she may end up being several inches shorter than before.

HRT can be taken in several ways: by pill; by a sticky plaster-type patch stuck to a fleshy area and replaced every three days; or by 'injected' pellets (implants), which last up to three months before they need re-placing.

Women who suffer from migraine may need to be carefully monitored if they want to begin HRT. In some cases it has been found that HRT can aggravate migraine, but other women have found it extremely helpful. One member of the British Migraine Association, writing in the association's newsletter, describes taking HRT as 'like waving a magic wand'. She says HRT has freed her from the perpetual fear of migraine as well as improving her general health because she no longer has to rely on analgesics to get by.

One disadvantage of HRT is that most women will have menstrual periods and even monthly breast tenderness. Some women may feel a little sick or get headaches during the first few weeks of treatment. Leg cramps are also quite common. These effects happen as your body adjusts to having a regular supply of hormones again, and usually disappear after a few weeks. But the advantages are stronger bones and muscles, better 'feeling' skin, the continuity of normal vaginal secretions, no hot flushes and a reduced risk of heart disease.

Studies show that both heart disease and female cancers of the uterus and ovaries are less frequent in women taking HRT. Because many, if not most, cancers of the breast can be treated by stopping a woman's body from producing oestrogen, or blocking its action, it has been suggested that HRT, which relies on oestrogen, could be a 'cause' of breast cancer. There is no evidence that is so, though expert researchers continue to debate the subject. The recommendation remains that for a fit woman, the advantages appear to heavily outweigh any potential disadvantages.

Beryl, a fifty-eight-year-old retired teacher, has endured migraine attacks all her life – and like many sufferers she has experienced them particularly before her periods, with patches of remission during pregnancy and after the menopause.

As a child I didn't realise I was suffering from migraine – I thought it was just travel sickness. When I got married I quickly became aware that stress triggered a migraine. I found, too, that alcohol would be a trigger. For years I thought it was white wine but any kind of dry wine affected me rather than a colour. Yet at other times I could get away with having a glass – the annoying thing was I could never tell when I would be able to get away with it.

I'd also have a migraine every month in the run up to my period, so premenstrual factors were definitely involved. At one stage I did try progesterone suppositories which helped a little and I was told about the importance of preventing low blood sugar levels when trying to alleviate the symptoms of premenstrual syndrome.

When I was pregnant I found that I didn't have the migraines as often. I'd heard that migraine can stop altogether during this time. They didn't stop for me but I only had about two or three attacks.

I'd always have a feeling before an attack. I knew there was no escape and that I was condemned to have a migraine. It's so hard to describe such a feeling – almost the beginnings of nausea, a pressure inside the head. Then I would be unable to digest any food. I could feel food sticking in my throat. I felt as if there was a blockage in the top half of my digestive system. The pain over my left eye would make me feel as if the eye was being gouged out. Then it would almost be a relief to vomit – it would be something to take my mind off the pain above my eye, even though vomiting itself would be so uncomfortable. Then I could retch on an empty stomach for anything up to twelve or more hours.

The pain would last twenty-four hours. It varied from twelve to twenty-four hours before it would seem to fade, which would be followed by a slight recurrence. So the attack could last thirty-six hours from the very beginning to the end.

It disrupted my life terribly. I would have to go to bed. My daughter, who is now grown up, says that when she was a child she hated coming home from school to find me stretched out on the sofa. She'd know immediately that she would have to look after herself. I had to lie on the sofa rather than go to bed, because at least it was downstairs and I could keep an eye on her. I hated having to do it but I had no choice.

I also felt terribly guilty when I had to let people down because of migraine. It also put a great strain on my marriage. My ex-husband, now late, was an alcoholic so there was already stress on the marriage without migraine. My present partner doesn't cause me any stress because he is so kind and he looks after me. So I wouldn't say migraine would cause as much strain on a good partnership.

Over the years Beryl has tried all manner of treatment from Cafergot suppositories, to Stemetil, to acupuncture, feverfew tablets and even dental treatment.

I have a wonderful GP who encourages me to try different things. When I retired from teaching two years ago I got a lump sum. So I went to a private dentist to get new crowns on my teeth. He measured my jaw and said that I had a badly arranged bite. He suggested I try an acrylic bite, which cost me £200, and it did work. I had to wear it all the time for the first six months and now I just wear it in bed at night. The idea is to realign my jaw so that my muscles get used to being in a different position and it helps to relieve tension in the back of my neck and shoulders.

It looks like a denture. It's pale pink plastic and it sits over the top of my bottom teeth. It's quite comfortable and you can eat while wearing it. It's brought my lower jaw forward and holds it in a position where it can't drop back.

Growing older has also meant a reduction in the frequency of Beryl's migraines.

They've started to diminish in the last couple of years. I had a hysterectomy at forty-nine and I'm not sure when my menopause started. I've tried HRT recently. My migraines stopped for about three months but then they came back once a month just as they used to. Without HRT my skin was beginning to lack lustre and I had no sex drive at all. My GP said he understood my reluctance not to carry on with it. I have changed types and now I'm not getting migraine, although if I feel one might be starting I immediately take a pink Migraleve and that does the trick every time.

MIGRAINE AND CHILDHOOD

Childhood migraine tends to be shorter than adult migraine. Often an attack can last just half an hour. The child usually looks pale, unwell and may have a fever. He or she may dislike bright lights and feel nauseous together with experiencing abdominal discomfort. In fact, stomach and other gastro-intestinal disturbances are more common symptoms than headaches in children. It's not unusual for a child with migraine to suffer from travel sickness, either.

Although childhood migraine may not last as long as an adult attack, for a child it can be just as difficult to cope with. Not only can their school time be interrupted, so too can play time which can result in a child feeling quite insecure and unhappy.

And migraine in a child can easily be disregarded or missed. The young child may not complain about a symptom, they may just go quiet and not seem able to explain what is wrong. If that is happening to your child it's well worth wondering if the cause could be migraine. If you are suspicious then a migraine clinic may be the best place to turn for the kind of specialist consultation that could make the diagnosis and so suggest a solution. I've heard it said that migraine that occurs in childhood has up to a fifty-fifty chance of going as the child grows – so there is every reason for hope.

A very common trigger factor in childhood migraine is not eating regularly and with not enough calories. Missing out on meals, which causes a low blood sugar level, as I've mentioned earlier, has been shown to play a part in migraine. Children very often don't eat all their meal, or don't want to eat, if something else is catching their attention. Then, in addition to this, they often race around using up lots of energy while they exercise, another common trigger factor. Experts now believe that children suffering from migraine can also be helped by making sure that they eat breakfast every day. If you think about it, a child who doesn't eat breakfast might have gone without food for more than twelve hours, especially if they had their last meal in the early evening.

It's essential too that if they don't have school meals at lunchtime, that their lunch box is packed with nutritious food and not just crisps and bars of chocolate!

Usually, treatment for a child with migraine will involve simple analgesics such as paracetemol and a lie down in a quiet, darkened room. In some cases preventative medicines may be prescribed. On no account give medicine you might have been prescribed for migraine to a child, or anyone else for that matter.

I'm often met with surprise when I talk about migraine in children – many people seem to think that it's just a problem encountered by adults. Yet when I've chatted to migraine sufferers about the history of their problem, with hindsight they can trace the headaches back to their childhood. Having thought about it, Albert, who's now a retired hotelier of sixty-nine, can remember suffering from migraine throughout his life.

> It seems as if I've had them for as long as I can remember. But if I think about it retrospectively, I'd say they must have started from about the age of four or five. Of course, in those days they weren't called migraines. I was told I was suffering from bilious attacks. I'd be sick frequently as a child and teenager, often it would be once a week.
>
> I'd never be given anything for them. I'd be put to bed and have to lie there until the attack passed. Looking back I can see now that sweet things triggered an attack. Bags of sweets and ice-cream were the main culprits. And, interestingly, when I was in the Army during the war, I was fairly free of migraines. Now I wonder whether that was something to do with not having a lot of sweet foods. In a way we had a very healthy diet during those years.

4: CONVENTIONAL TREATMENT

Many migraine sufferers don't always seek treatment, for a variety of reasons such as they don't want to bother the doctor, they feel they'll just be told to take paracetamol and give up cheese and chocolate which they've already done, or because they have encountered unhelpful advice on previous occasions. My advice is, *don't give up*. Make it clear to your doctor just how bad your symptoms are when the over-the-counter medicines or your usual means of relief aren't working. If needs be, request a second opinion.

Your doctor may decide to refer you to a hospital neurology department at one of the many hospitals nationwide which have a particular interest in dealing with migraine. Some hospitals even have specialist clinics, such as the Princess Margaret Migraine Clinic in West London, and there's also, of course, the City of London Migraine Clinic. At hospital, specialist tests may sometimes be done to rule out the possibility of more serious conditions or abnormalities, or to measure the electrical activity of the brain.

Generally speaking, however, painkillers such as aspirin or paracetamol (see also page 87) are enough to ease a mild attack. One option open to your doctor is short-term (also known as acute) treatment, by prescribing drugs to be taken when a migraine attack is underway.

ACUTE TREATMENT

Ergotamine

Ergotamine is useful for sufferers (excluding children) who find that simple analgesics don't help at all. But on no account take more than your doctor or pharmacist tells you to. It can be prescribed in tablet form or by suppository (Cafergot). You may even be prescribed an inhaler, like Medihaler Ergotamine, which contains ergotamine tartrate.

Ergotamine aborts attacks of migraine by its specific vasoconstrictor – arterial narrowing – effect on over-widened or widening arteries outside the skull. Cafergot also contains caffeine to enhance absorption and the suppositories are thought to be most useful for people who have nausea and vomiting quite early in the migraine attack and therefore cannot 'keep anything down', including tablets. So, as with any medicine for migraine, you do need to take ergotamine tablets as early as possible in the attack.

One or two Cafergot tablets taken at the first sign of a migraine are usually enough to bring some relief. Some people might need a higher dose but you should never take more than four tablets (which is equivalent to 4 milligrams of ergotamine) in a twenty-four-hour period. And you should really use the lowest dose possible to bring about an easing of the pain. You shouldn't take more than eight tablets during the course of a week and, according to the manufacturers Sandoz, there should be an interval of at least four days between successive days' doses.

Lingraine contains ergotamine and the tablets are designed for sublingual administration – to be placed under the tongue. One tablet is to be taken at the first sign of an attack to be repeated after thirty minutes. However, you must not take more than three tablets in twenty-four hours, and no more than six in a week.

Migril contains ergotamine, cyclizine hydrochloride (an antihistamine for the nausea) and caffeine, and again is prescribed for the relief of an acute migraine. The usual dose is one tablet at the first warning of an attack. If needed, half or one tablet can be additionally taken at half-hourly intervals. No more than four tablets should be taken in any one attack (8 milligrams). And no more than six tablets should be taken in any one week.

Medihaler Ergotamine contains a suspension of ergotamine in an aerosol propellant for the rapid relief of migraine. Micronised ergotamine tartrate taken by inhalation is rapidly absorbed from the blood-rich lining of the breathing tubes into the body's bloodstream. Advantages of taking the drug this way is the speed with which it's absorbed, the fact that the drug isn't 'interfered with' first within the digestive tract or the liver (so a lower dose can be used) and that the drug is kept in the body despite vomiting. One inhalation should be taken at the first sign of an attack and should be repeated if necessary after five minutes. No more than six inhalations should be taken in any twenty-four-hour period and no more than fifteen in one week.

If you experience tingling, numbness or coldness in the fingers or toes, you should stop taking ergotamine and consult your doctor as soon as possible. This is because its effects may be over-constricting your blood vessels and it's likely that your doctor will tell you to stop taking the tablets or reduce the dose. Other side-effects can include nausea, vomiting, drowsiness, confusion and dizziness – often symptoms of the migraine which can make it difficult to determine whether they're caused by the attack itself or the drug. Long-term use of ergotamine can result in a rebound-type headache. This means that when you stop taking the tablets the symptoms not only return but do so in an even more unpleasant way. Other medicines can do this as well – for example, when the older type of tranquillisers that were taken for anxiety were stopped suddenly, the anxiety returned even worse than it had been in the first place.

Ergotamine shouldn't be used as a prophylactic – preventative – medicine because of the risk of inducing ergotism. This is, as mentioned above, when the medicine over-constricts the blood vessels. Though rare, with a heavy overdose the vessels may constrict so much that the blood supply to the fingers and toes is cut off, and the tissues are damaged as a result, sometimes severely.

Non-Steroidal Anti-Inflammatory Drugs

Some sufferers have been prescribed NSAIDs – Non-Steroidal Anti-Inflammatory Drugs – medicines commonly taken by arthritis sufferers. Usually they are not formally recognised as having a role to play in migraine, but as a one-off have been found to be useful. They are usually available in suppository form and most are only available on prescription.

There are many types of non-steroidal anti-inflammatory drugs available. They work by inhibiting the production of prostaglandins, which pass on pain signals to the brain. Examples are naproxen and mefenamic acid. The most common side-effects of non-steroidal anti-inflammatory drugs include nausea, vomiting, heartburn or indigestion. Naproxen can cause gastrointestinal disorders, as can mefenamic acid.

Midrid

Midrid, which contains isometheptene mucate and paracetamol, can provide fast relief of migraine headaches which stem from dilated cranial vessels. Isometheptene mucate constricts the blood vessels within the brain and the paracetamol acts as a painkiller. Short-lived dizziness can be a side-effect of these capsules.

Imigran

Another prescription medicine used to treat attacks as they occur is Imigran, and as it is the newest of the migraine medicines, I feel it is worth a detailed mention here.

Imigran is currently being used in around twenty-two countries worldwide as a treatment for acute migraine attacks. Glaxo Pharmaceuticals spent twenty years and £130 million on developing the drug and its arrival was long awaited by the many migraine sufferers I know.

The product contains sumatriptan, the first of a new group of medicines developed for the treatment of migraine. As the symptoms may be due to swollen blood vessels around the brain which then pinch nearby nervous pathways thus causing pain, medicines like Imigran probably work by reducing the size of these blood vessels and are called '5HT1 agonists'. It is the fact that Imigran causes only the *cranial* blood vessels to constrict rather than blood vessels throughout the body that makes it such a breakthrough.

The British Migraine Association was keen to discover just how their members had got on with this new treatment and they received more than 250 letters. Interestingly, 85 per cent of those who wrote found Imigran, in either injection or tablet form, successful. Fifteen per cent found it didn't help them at all, and a similar percentage were refused it on prescription – there have been worries about the drug's cost. (It costs the NHS just over £20 per injection and the tablets around £45 for a pack of six.)

But I have to say that although some people have found that this new drug has not helped them, many migraine sufferers have described it as an absolute miracle which has thankfully transformed their lives. As migraine can mean misery for millions of people it is comforting to hear news like this.

Maureen, a forty-eight-year-old bookkeeper, has suffered from migraine for twenty-two years, and has been fortunate enough to have some success with Imigran.

When I have a migraine it feels as though somebody is tying the blood vessels in my head in knots. I'm incapable of doing anything. Sometimes the migraine will last twenty-four hours, often forty-eight hours, and all I can do is stay in bed. I can't eat and can't really sleep.

There was no set pattern but I'm sure they were linked to periods. I knew there would usually be one week in a month when I would be OK but the rest of the time I couldn't really plan ahead because I'd never know when migraine would strike.

Like so many sufferers, Maureen refused to let migraine totally dominate her life. And, again like so many other people, there were times when she found that easier to say than carry out.

I did try very hard not to let migraine rule my life. Yet no matter how hard I tried there were times when I had to cancel nights out at the last minute because I'd think I'd be fine the next day, I'll make myself better. But you can't. Of course, then I would feel guilty that I'd let other people down. Not that people have been unsympathetic but I do get the impression that people who've never had migraine don't really understand that it's more than just a headache and that you can't carry on as normal.

Maureen had tried various medicines in the past without much luck, most often preferring to buy Migraleve (see page 89) from the pharmacist, 'Although I didn't like taking them that often because they would make me so drowsy.' She first found out about Imigran from the City of London Migraine Clinic.

I know it sounds ridiculous but when I first heard about it, only the auto-injectors were available and I thought I couldn't try it because I do have a fear of injections. I thought I couldn't possibly inject myself. People told me it couldn't be worse than having a migraine so I thought I'd give it a try. I had two auto-injectors and I've still got one in the drawer.

On this particular day I knew my headache was developing into a migraine so I got out the auto-injector and sat with it against my leg for about fifteen minutes and I thought I just can't do it.

I tried to psyche myself up and told myself not to be so ridiculous. I eventually had a go but didn't do it properly and all the Imigran ran down my leg – and I ended up in bed for two days with a migraine. Not even the prospect of two days in agony could make me do it. I know it sounds daft.

Maureen is not alone. Many otherwise brave men and women can keel over at the very thought of an injection. I've seen it happen in the forces when the men needed to be injected one after the other on first entering the service.

When Imigran became available in tablet form, Maureen's run of luck changed.

I found that Imigran helped me even when my migraine had taken quite a hold – when a normal tablet would have no chance of giving me any relief. I couldn't believe it. I've found that within an hour the pain just suddenly goes away. It's marvellous.

Like so many sufferers, Maureen has found that she's been able to prevent further migraine bouts by taking a tablet when she feels an attack developing. She's noticed a couple of minor side-effects but her main problem is a GP who's beginning to complain about the cost of prescribing Imigran.

After I've taken Imigran I find that if I have a hot drink, such as a cup of tea, my throat burns. Another consequence is that if I put my hands in hot water, the temperature feels a lot hotter than it actually is. But these side-effects aren't a problem, especially as I know what they are. [Goodness knows why Maureen has experienced these symptoms as they are not to be expected.] My main problem is my GP who has complained that I've already cost him a lot of money, about £500 so far. He's wanted me to try cheaper medicines I haven't taken before, but I'm not prepared to give something up when I know it works so well. I can't say I like taking drugs but when you've found something that helps, you don't want to be without it.

Anne, a forty-one-year-old part-time adult literacy tutor, describes Imigran as an absolute miracle. She's suffered from migraine for twenty-four years, the attacks increasing in severity with her age. There is no definite pattern to them and she's found that migraine has severely interrupted her life at times, especially when her two children were small.

I think my migraines are more likely around my time of the month but they could strike at any time really. If I drank red wine I would have a headache not long after and by the next morning I would have to be flat on my back in bed – in fact, it's now fifteen years since I've touched any wine.

The pain of an attack doesn't make it worth it. It's so severe, on the right-hand side of my head from my temple down to the cheekbone, all I want is for somebody to remove the right half of my head. The pain is horrendous, worse than toothache, far, far worse.

I have to stay in bed all day – from twelve to twenty-four hours. I'd try to sleep as much as I could, but you can't sleep for twenty-four hours. And I'd have to be totally in the dark. I couldn't keep any food down. When I visited a hospital migraine clinic they reckoned that my stomach had stopped working before my headache became apparent to me and that's why it was impossible to keep anything down. I couldn't drink even a glass of water so I'd become very dehydrated. When it cleared I'd always long for a glass of fizzy lemonade. Then it would take another twenty-four hours for my system to settle down and often I could be out of action for a total of three days.

Fortunately I have a wonderful husband who has been very supportive. But when my two children were babies it was so difficult I had to rely on a good friend to help out. She used to suffer from tension headaches and was sympathetic, so when I had a migraine she would have the children for the day. Often we have to phone round and ask friends to pick up the children from school. It makes me feel as though I have to pay everybody back all the time. So when anyone asks a favour I always say yes because I never know when I might have to call on them to return it and ask them to look after the children. But since I've discovered Imigran it looks as if my days of relying on other people are over.

I'm also lucky to have an excellent GP who is willing for me to try different things. I have in the past found a lot of doctors quite unsympathetic to migraine sufferers. I even had one who told me that he had migraine and nothing could be done for him so why should he try to do something for me!

I first tried the auto-injector, although the first time I couldn't do it and my husband had to do it for me. I don't know why – I'm quite used to it now even though it stings quite a lot. If I wake in the early morning with a migraine attack developing my husband will give me an injection usually at about five in the morning. It helps then if I move around as normal by about seven. If I just lie there I feel worse. If I keep going the migraine clears up.

I've also used the tablets too. Imigran works for me every time. It varies in how long it takes to be effective, sometimes it's eased my pain in about ten minutes, at other times it can take an hour or so. Sometimes I don't feel 100 per cent afterwards, perhaps a little under the weather and a bit tired. Or as if I'm not quite with the world. I do get a funny taste in my mouth, a kind of dryness at the back of my throat. But I couldn't care less about that.

The new medicine has honestly changed our lives considerably. I feel Imigran has given me three extra days every month for living, not just existing. I can now plan things without having to worry – things like going away on holiday. At last we can say 'yes' to everything. It's made us both more carefree. We've gone out and done lots of things together, going to the cinema without having to cancel, for example. That alone has made a difference to our marriage, even though my husband has always been so understanding. Looking back at some of my boyfriends, I don't think they would have been as understanding as the one I decided to marry. In fact, my husband has often taken time off work to help out when I've been ill. He's said that taking time off is irrelevant compared to what I've been through.

As is to be expected, not everyone has tried Imigran with such positive results. Both Beryl (who talks about her migraines on page 46) and Charlotte (on page 112) were bitterly disappointed that Imigran did not make them feel any better. In fact, Beryl discovered that the drug made her almost feel worse.

I tried the auto-injector, which hurt like hell, and found that my migraine hadn't really gone away – and I was truly confident that it was going to work. I felt some pressure diminishing but the nausea was the worst I have ever had. I was sick for three days and it took me the rest of the week to recover. I didn't ask my GP for any more – I didn't want to feel like that ever again. I was terribly disappointed because I was so eager to try it.

If Imigran does work for you, or you would like to try it, don't be misled into thinking that the drug can be used preventatively. It can treat an acute attack, but bear in mind that if you do know what triggers your migraine, and you are able to avoid these triggers, you still need to do so. The British Migraine Association also points out that migraine sufferers should be aware that Imigran should not be taken less than seventy-two hours after ergotamine and ergotamine preparations should not be taken less than twelve hours after Imigran. This is because both drugs affect the blood vessels.

Most people taking this medicine seem to find that it

causes no problems. But if any of the following side-effects occur you should check with your doctor: sudden wheeziness; fluttering or tightness in the chest; swelling of eyelids, face or lips; a skin rash. These symptoms could mean that you are allergic to the medicine. Other side-effects include tiredness, dizziness, flushing, feelings of tingling, warmth, heaviness, pressure, tightness or sometimes pain in different parts of the body, including the chest and throat, weakness, and nausea or vomiting when not part of a migraine attack. These are not usually very troublesome and pass off with time.

Anti-nausea drugs

Products containing anti-nausea drugs (Migravess, Migravess Forte, Paramax or Maxolon and Primperan) can also be helpful in dealing with migraine.

Migravess is an analgesic and anti-emetic (prevents nausea and vomiting) for the quick relief of headache and nausea associated with migraine. The tablets contain metoclopramide monohydrochloride, aspirin, sodium bicarbonate and citric acid. Two tablets are dissolved in water and should be taken at the first sign of an attack. No more than three doses are to be taken per twenty-four hours.

Paramax combines metoclopramide with paracetamol – the paracetamol will relieve pain and the metoclopramide will encourage a rapid absorption. Metoclopramide, in line with other anti-emetic drugs, can cause drowsiness, lethargy, dizziness, insomnia, diarrhoea and flatulence.

Maxolon, Primperan or Metromid (metoclopramide hydrochloride) may be prescribed to help the symptoms of nausea and vomiting, and to overcome gastric stasis – the stopping of the stomach's digestive movements – associated with attacks of migraine. The improvement in gastric emptying, once the movements occur normally again, assists the absorption of concurrently administered oral anti-migraine medicines which may otherwise be impaired in such patients.

Stemetil, Buccastem or Vertigon are other prescription medicines which can help reduce the nausea and vomiting associated with migraine. These medicines contain prochlorperazine maleate, a potent phenothiazine treatment which is also used in the treatment of certain forms of mental illness, unrelated to its benefits for the migraine sufferer. It can cause drowsiness, dizziness, a dry mouth, insomnia, agitation and mild skin reactions.

Motilium is another given to ease nausea and vomiting. This medicine contains domperidone maleate, a dopamine antagonist – in other words, it counteracts dopamine, one of the brain chemicals.

Prochlorperazine and domperidone work by blocking certain chemical receptors in the brain, known to trigger the vomiting reflex.

PROPHYLACTICS

If migraine attacks are very frequent, your doctor may prescribe long-term preventative treatment, also known as prophylactic treatment. This could be one of the drugs often used to control high blood pressure, a beta-blocker such as Betaloc, Betaloc SA, Lopresor or Lopresor SR. Such medicines have an effect upon the blood vessels. Others include Corgard (Nadolol), Inderal, Inderal LA/Half-Inderal LA (propranolol hydrochloride) and Blocadren (timolol maleate). Migraine occurs as the arteries to the brain first 'close' and then open and beta-blockers have been found to dampen this process. Side-effects of these drugs can include mild dizziness and mild stomach upsets.

Clonidine (Dixarit), which is also used for meno-pausal flushing, may be prescribed though is not used quite so frequently these days because it seems to be less effective than pizotifen (see below) or beta-blockers. Treatment with Dixarit diminishes the responsiveness of peripheral vessels to constrictor and dilator stimuli, thereby preventing the vascular changes associated with migraine. Side-effects can include sedation or, initially, a dry mouth. Dizziness, nausea and unsettled nights have also been reported.

Then there is Sanomigran, which contains the anti-histamine pizotifen (a drug related to some of the anti-depressants). It is also a serotinin antagonist (explained on page 65). The medicine is used to prevent migraine headaches or reduce their frequency and severity, but should be taken regularly and usually for at least four months. This drug is sometimes used to help childhood migraine. The prophylactic effect is associated with its ability to modify the chemical changes that accompany a headache. The medicine can make people drowsy, cause dizziness, sickness or cause an increase in appetite or weight gain. If you take Sanomigran you can avoid putting on weight either by taking it at night or by trying not to pick at food throughout the day. Although any extra weight gained is normally lost fairly quickly once treatment is stopped.

Many people find Sanomigran helpful. Katherine, the journalist I mentioned earlier, who regularly had weekend headaches once the pressure of her working week was off, tried taking Sanomigran for four months, with great success.

My doctor was very sympathetic when I went to see her about my recurring headaches after lots of sarcastic remarks at work about my migraine. Sometimes a particularly bad headache would last until Monday and now and again I did have to have the day off – although I nearly always did some work at home in that case. I felt too guilty to do nothing.

But you'd think that my boss, a woman who also suffered from migraine, would show some understanding but she didn't. I'm sure she thought that if she could cope and carry on working hard in the office so could I. Luckily my doctor was extremely helpful. She immediately told me that my headaches were definitely migraine and that the pattern of headaches developing as the stress was over was quite a common one. She also said she had just the thing to help me.

I'd never heard of prophylactic treatment for migraine. But she explained the need for this type of treatment by saying that my body had to be re-educated as to how it should behave. Although I wasn't too keen on taking drugs for an extended period of time, this explanation seemed to make sense to me and I thought it was worth trying. By this time I was really fed up of my migraines.

The funny thing is that by now I was more worried about what other people thought of me than I was about suffering such discomfort every week. Because I either had a headache on a Friday evening or a Saturday evening, I was constantly having to cancel nights out. My boyfriend was very understanding because he knew that I have quite a high tolerance for pain and that if I say I'm in pain, then I really must be. He didn't mind staying in at the weekend.

Sometimes I felt that I just couldn't cancel an arrangement, say for the second weekend in a row, so I would go and try to put on a brave face while the right half of my head was pulsating. Sometimes I found it very difficult to keep track of people's conversations. Concentration was impossible. I'm sure that often people who didn't know me very well must have thought I was quite a vague kind of person, who always seemed to be thinking about something else when they spoke to me. Just trying to sit out a migraine in such circumstances was nothing less than torture at times. It would be even worse if we were in a restaurant which was smoky, and other women at the table would be drenched in perfume as well. Very often I would end up just pushing the food around my plate to make it look as if I had eaten something. It was hell. And it was supposed to be my weekend break!

Katherine took one Sanomigran every evening about an hour before she went to bed as her doctor had warned her that the treatment could cause drowsiness.

I did find that initially I would still feel drowsy in the morning, as if I was drugged. I would sleep throughout my fifty-minute train journey to work, although by the time I got to the office I felt quite lively and normal. This side-effect seemed to wear off after about a month, or maybe I just got used to feeling that way in the morning, I can't say for definite. I don't remember any other side-effects. I do remember that the treatment seemed to affect my migraines quite dramatically. I did have a headache that first weekend but it wasn't as bad as it usually was, and each subsequent weekend the headaches became less and less severe until I didn't have one any more. It's difficult to pinpoint exactly how long it took for my migraines to clear up because it was a gradual effect. But by the time I stopped taking Sanomigran four months later I had got myself out of a vicious cycle of expecting to have a migraine each weekend – and suddenly I started to enjoy life again.

Another medicine used in the prophylactic treatment of migraine is Deseril, which contains methysergide maleate, a potent serotonin antagonist. Serotonin is an enzyme involved in the vascular changes which produce headaches. The minimum effective dose should be used – which is often a dose that will stop about three-quarters of attacks rather than *all* headaches. The most commonly reported side-effects are nausea, heartburn, abdominal discomfort, vomiting, dizziness, tiredness and drowsiness. Because of these, Deseril should only be taken under hospital supervision.

Periactin (cyproheptadine hydrochloride) is another medicine which dampens the automatic effects that occur in the brain and local tissues in the early stages of migraine – that is, it is a serotonin and histamine antagonist with anticholinergic and sedative properties. An anticholinergic chemical is one that prevents the passage of impulses down 'reflex' nerve pathways in the body and so can relieve symptoms or produce a beneficial effect. This medicine can cause drowsiness.

Diuretics are sometimes helpful for women whose attacks are linked to their menstrual cycle. As is pyridoxine, vitamin B6.

Period-time migraines often respond to treatment with the hormone progesterone. Pessaries containing progesterone (Cyclogest, for example) can be prescribed for premenstrual syndrome – and quite often women who find their migraines are linked to their monthly cycle do experience other premenstrual symptoms too. These pessaries are suitable for vaginal or rectal insertion, usually beginning on the fourteenth day of the cycle and continuing treatment until onset of menstruation. If you use barrier methods of contraception then the pessaries should be inserted rectally. Sometimes periods can start earlier than expected as a result of this treatment – or, more rarely, they may be delayed. Soreness, diarrhoea and flatulence can occur with rectal administration.

Tablets such as Menzol, or Primolut N (norethisterone), for example, can ease premenstrual symptoms such as headache, migraine, breast discomfort, water retention, tachycardia and psychological disturbances. You will be advised to take a tablet two to three times a day from the nineteenth to the twenty-sixth day of the cycle, and treatment should be repeated for several cycles. When treatment is stopped, you may find you remain symptom-free for a number of months. Side-effects of this type of treatment are not that frequent at standard doses – the commonest is breakthrough bleeding (bleeding or spotting during the month when you don't have your period or it isn't due) particularly when treatment is continuous over a long period. Other reported effects include nausea, vomiting, acne, oedema, weight gain, headache and depression.

SOME GENERAL TIPS ABOUT MIGRAINE MEDICINE

■ Remember that when your doctor hands you a prescription for migraine with your name at the top, he or she means it to be taken by *you alone* – and not a fellow sufferer. It's designed to deal with your specific problem, not any symptoms of your husband, wife, neighbour or friend. So don't dish out medicines, and don't accept any from anyone else either – no matter how well meaning the person is.

■ Always remind your doctor if you already have a medical condition when you are being prescribed a medicine – for example, if you have asthma, diabetes, any allergies (aspirin intolerance, for instance), heart disease, high blood pressure and so on.

■ If you are pregnant, even if you only think you might be, always tell your doctor. Some medicines may be harmful – particularly if taken during the first twelve weeks of pregnancy; or often there is just inadequate evidence of safety in human pregnancy. Some medicines also may not be safe to take while you are breastfeeding so always tell your doctor if you are.

■ Along with its needed effects, a medicine may cause side-effects, as I have already mentioned. You should always discuss side-effects with your doctor or pharmacist, or if you feel unwell or have any unusual discomfort after taking your medicine.

■ Almost all medicines and pills will do you harm if taken in too great a quantity or incorrectly. So follow the instructions on the label. Twice the amount won't do you twice as much good, or work any quicker, and could be dangerous.

■ Never take another analgesic within four hours of having taken the first, even if it is of a different type or brand, unless instructed to do so by your doctor.

■ Tablets or capsules can stick in your throat, so take them with plenty of water while sitting or standing up. Swallow capsules whole, unless you are told to open them. Soluble tablets should be dissolved in a tumblerful of water.

■ Some medicines may cause drowsiness. If affected don't drive or operate machinery and avoid alcoholic drink. Alcohol may change the way your medicine works.

■ Never put your tablets into another smaller bottle – always keep medicines in their original containers so you know the labelling is accurate.

■ If you accidentally take an overdose of your medicine, either get in touch with your doctor immediately, or go to your nearest hospital casualty department. Always take any remaining tablets, the container and the label with you, so that the medicines can be identified correctly.

■ If you have been prescribed medication for migraine, I would recommend that you always keep it with you. That way, wherever you are, you will be able to take your medication at the first sign of an attack. Taking anti-migraine medication as soon as you feel an attack developing is one way to shorten the attack's duration.

I'm often asked by people whether it's worth bothering their doctor, especially if their symptoms turn out to be the result of something inconsequential, and particularly if it's 'just a headache'. But I would say that if you are worried about something you should always check it out. As people don't normally have any medical training, the only practical criterion you can apply when deciding whether or not to go to the doctor is your own unease and worry.

Your doctor can then either recommend investigation or treatment for worrying new symptoms, or reassure you that there's nothing to be concerned about. Such reassurance for patients is a very straightforward matter and part of a doctor's job, a part that should save you – and him or her – time in the long run.

DENTAL HELP

Finally, some experts believe that a percentage of migraine sufferers clench their teeth while they're sleeping. It's thought that this could cause jaw spasms which might trigger migraine when they wake up. A splint worn over the back teeth could stop this problem. Other dental theories include badly aligned teeth and an imbalance in the bite, which can lead to muscle strain. While wearing a dentist-recommended splint may put this right, a form of jaw physiotherapy called bite rehabilitation can also bring benefits.

5: ALTERNATIVE TREATMENT

People still say to me, 'Doctors don't believe in alternative medicine.' Well, here's one who does – but it does depend on what you mean by alternative (or complementary) medicine and what you expect from it.

No responsible alternative practitioner – for example, an acupuncturist, homoeopath or naturopath (a therapist who uses no drugs, just natural 'forces' like foods, heat, light and gentle massage) – would suggest that they have the treatment and the cure for all human ills. If someone is badly injured in a road accident only an experienced surgeon has the varied skills required to repair the injuries and save life. On the other hand, a sufferer will sometimes be helped by an alternative practitioner after his or her many symptoms have been fully investigated by all the latest medical diagnostic procedures, and no abnormality other than the symptoms themselves has been discovered.

Trying 'alternative' treatments like acupuncture, for instance, is something I would recommend to anyone who has found no joy through traditional methods of coping with migraine. You may find that the only thing that is affected is your wallet, but on the other hand you may gain valuable relief and that in itself is usually worth any money you might have to pay out. There is indeed, these days, a growing acknowledgement of the benefits of osteopathy, chiropractic and acupuncture and other alternative therapies. Earlier this year there was even an announcement that a Chair of Complementary Medicine is to be installed at Exeter University.

But I would advise caution. Make sure that if you are

going to give one of these treatments a try that the specialist you see is appropriately qualified. You can always ask your doctor, or friends who have found the treatment beneficial, to recommend someone. Give them a go but don't spend a fortune persevering with treatments for the sake of it if you find that you are getting no favourable results.

ACUPUNCTURE

You could not be blamed for wondering why acupuncture seems to have such a surprising success rate for so many completely different ailments and diseases. The reason is that it's not just some ancient superstition that's now available to desperate people as a last resort. It works by triggering the brain to secrete its own chemicals, which function rather like natural painkillers or tranquillisers, so providing relief for sufferers of all types of problems.

Acupuncture itself is no newcomer to complementary medicine. It has been around as a form of treatment in China for five thousand years and these days more and more people in the West are turning to it for a wide variety of ills.

When I discuss acupuncture I am constantly asked, what is the theory behind it, what does it actually involve and how can it help me? So I'll try to explain. Traditional acupuncture is a 'holistic' form of medicine – a philosophy which not only treats the symptom but also aims to improve the total well-being of the person. Practitioners believe that many physical conditions can be aggravated by, or even be due to, emotional stress, unsuitable diet and other factors. So your first visit to an acupuncturist will probably include detailed questions about your lifestyle and a thorough examination

– the tongue is especially important in making a diagnosis so don't be surprised if this is carefully examined!

Acupuncture aims to correct any disharmony within the body – to achieve a balance between positive and negative energy which the Chinese call Yin and Yang. An imbalance, they say, leads to disease. This energy flows along pathways in the body called 'meridians'. These cannot be seen but can be detected using special techniques and can be likened to the nerve pathways known to Western doctors. There are twelve main meridians either side of the body, each related to specific organs such as the heart, liver and stomach. There are also other meridians, such as those used when treating emotional problems like depression and nervousness. Twelve different pulses on the wrists also relate to the various organs and these, too, are taken into account when the acupuncturist is deciding on treatment.

Each meridian has many points along it in precise positions called 'acupoints'. During acupuncture very fine needles are inserted into several of these points, carefully chosen depending on the problem being treated. This is said to feel no worse than an accidental pin-prick and probably about eight needles will be used though it may be anything from one to twenty. They are inserted to varying depths, twirled from time to time and usually left in place for about twenty minutes each session.

At first it is surprising that the needles are often inserted in places that appear unrelated to the position of the pain or the symptoms. This is because the points on the meridians can affect parts of the body some distance away and many points interrelate. The outer ear, for example, has a large number of acupoints which correspond to various parts of the body. Sometimes the needles will be slightly heated to add to their effect.

Electroacupuncture is often used for shorter periods of time. The needles are similar but rather than being manipulated by hand they are made to vibrate by an electric current from a machine known as an acupunctoscope.

Many studies now show that acupuncture can relieve a wide variety of symptoms and can also help problems such as obesity, giving up smoking and reducing the craving for alcohol and drugs. It is thought to relieve pain partly by stimulating the body's production of natural painkillers called endorphins – in tests raised levels have been detected twenty minutes after treatment. We know that it can also have a calming effect on an overactive gut and using specific acupuncture points on the back has been shown to enlarge the breathing tubes and may help in asthma and chronic bronchitis. Other conditions that can benefit include skin problems, back pain, arthritis, insomnia, anxiety and depression, but no one can predict who will respond and who will not.

Acupuncture tends to work in stages. Often the first visit is ineffective but there should be progressive improvement after that. A course of treatment usually involves four to ten sessions and the effect can last six to nine months – sometimes longer. Occasional sessions may then be needed to maintain the benefit.

Always be sure to go to a well-qualified acupuncturist – those with letters after their name such as BAAR or TAS. Any adverse effects should then be most unlikely and you can be sure that the needles used will be properly sterilised.

Sometimes acupuncture can be used in conjunction with conventional medicine to improve the patient's general well-being. There are some practitioners – many GPs, for instance – who have done a shortened course in acupuncture, not involving the whole philosophy, and will use it in a limited way, such as to relieve pain.

Sufferers seem to have different experiences of acupuncture. Sheila, a thirty-six-year-old single parent, who talks about the other self-help measures she takes on page 96, found that acupuncture aided relaxation, which she believes was a beneficial thing in itself.

It did help me relax but I was very psyched up about acupuncture. I really wanted it to help and believed that it would. But as I'm on social security I couldn't afford to go on with the £15 sessions for very long. I did spend about £300 over six months and the treatment did help a bit. I would have carried on paying for more treatment if I'd had the money. I found the treatment gave me peace of mind. In my opinion peace of mind helps you cope with pain, even if it doesn't ease it.

HERBAL REMEDIES

A book on migraine wouldn't be complete without a mention of one fairly popular herbal remedy. Recent research has shown that a daily dose of a humble plant called feverfew (it looks like a miniature chrysanthemum and is now sold by many nursery gardens – the botanical name for the variety of feverfew you need is *Tanacetum parthenium*) helps many people to control their migraine by reducing the intensity of their headache and easing the nausea and vomiting. Possibly as many as seven out of ten sufferers find relief.

But how does it work, you may ask? Well, the active ingredients are thought to be chemical compounds which go to work on platelets. These are small cells which circulate in the blood and can clump together to act like natural 'sand bags' as they block any bleeding caused by an injury. These compounds help prevent a hormone called serotonin being released from the platelets. Some people believe that serotonin plays a part in migraine attacks by reducing blood flow to the brain.

It's also been recently reported in an issue of *Migraine News* that research to measure the amounts of parthenolide, the substance thought to be responsible for feverfew's ability to prevent migraine, has been carried out at University Hospital in Nottingham. The philosophy behind herbal medicine is that it is usually better to take the whole part of the plant – in this case the actual leaves – rather than just the active ingredient. However, the leaves do contain naturally high levels of parthenolide, in any case. Two or three leaves can be eaten in a sandwich sweetened with a little honey because it does have quite a bitter taste, and feverfew capsules and tablets are available from some pharmacies and health food shops.

You shouldn't take feverfew if you are pregnant or while breastfeeding and a minority of sufferers have found that it can give them mouth ulcers. For products available over-the-counter, see page 90.

HOMOEOPATHIC REMEDIES

Homoeopathy is said to be a completely safe form of therapy and homoeopathic medicines are even available under the National Health Service. This form of treatment is relatively new in comparison with acupuncture – it was first developed nearly two hundred years ago by a German physician, scholar and chemist, Samuel Hahnemann, out of the principle that 'like cures like'. Symptoms are treated by giving a minute dose of a substance which if given in larger quantities to a healthy person will actually *cause* those symptoms. Even in conventional medicine this principle is sometimes used – for instance, controlled doses of radiation are given to cure cancer, which can in turn be caused by too much radiation.

Homoeopathists believe in the body's natural ability to heal itself. A homoeopath will therefore aim to give a remedy which will encourage this process of stimulating the body's natural forces of recovery – unlike a conventional doctor who prescribes medicines to suppress symptoms (aspirin, for instance, to bring down a temperature, or antihistamines to dry up a runny nose).

Many homoeopaths are qualified doctors who have done a further year's training in homoeopathy. They may become GPs or work in homoeopathic hospitals (there are about six of these in the UK) and their treatment is available on the NHS or privately. The advantage of consulting a medically qualified homoeopath is that they are trained in diagnosis. If you do consult a homoeopath who is not also a doctor, make sure he or she has done a full homoeopathic training at an approved college.

Obviously, homoeopathy isn't going to help everyone, and some people are very sceptical about it. But if it does help – especially if it's in the hands of a responsible professional – it must be good.

There are remedies available over-the-counter (see page 90) but it is a fundamental principle of homoeopathy that the remedy should be tailor-made for the person, not the disorder.

ALEXANDER TECHNIQUE

The Alexander Technique is a gentle method aimed at relaxing muscles and improving posture by undoing bad sitting and standing habits. The technique was first developed in the 1890s by Frederick Matthias Alexander, an Australian actor and reciter. He became hoarse during performances and so worked out a new approach to balance, posture and movement which resulted in a great improvement in his general health.

His technique is a gentle one which helps to relax muscles by teaching the pupil to sit, stand and move gracefully without strain. In this way, so the theory goes, you can rid yourself of the persistent tension that so often causes a variety of problems, particularly headaches, backache, tiredness and depression. Many dance and drama schools teach the technique and it's even become popular in sport – the 1990 World Cup Italian football team is said to have used it in training.

The technique teaches you to listen to your body and helps you find ways to change your posture to avoid effort that just isn't necessary and to stop you slipping back into your old habits of slouching or hunching your shoulders or pulling your head back needlessly. Many people push out their jaw and stretch their neck when getting up from a sitting position instead of using their leg muscles to push themselves up. Other bad habits can be drawing your chin towards your chest, rounding your shoulders and, at the same time, almost trying to make your body appear shorter. It's surprising how many people do this when they're feeling anxious, or stiffen all their muscles without even knowing it. The technique helps you understand when you are working against your natural poise and allowing your bad habits to take over. It teaches you how to put this understanding into practice, especially when you're under stress.

An Alexander Technique teacher can point out to you tension you weren't even aware of and how you trigger this tension at the thought of movement. The teacher then instructs you on how to prevent this. Most importantly the technique improves your awareness of your body so that you can recognise tension before it builds to the point of causing muscle pain.

It's very difficult to get across exactly how the technique works and if you are interested it is possibly worth trying a lesson or two to understand what all the fuss is about. Some people find one lesson so relaxing they want to learn more about the technique in order to adapt its teachings into their everyday life.

The Alexander Technique is taught on a one-to-one basis because the teacher needs to place his or her hands on the pupil's body as well as explaining the method. Also, different people have different bad habits so treatment needs to be designed to your individual lifestyle. The teacher usually chooses a simple movement, say sitting or standing, to work on. Some time is also spent lying on a table while you are taught how to perfect the technique.

It's beneficial to begin with two or three lessons a week, gradually spacing them out as you acquire the ability to practise on your own. You can discuss alternatives with the teacher if this is impractical. If it does appeal to you, it's generally accepted that you'll need a course of twenty to thirty lessons. Some local authority education centres run group classes. The cost of a lesson is comparable to a session with an osteopath, acupuncturist or other alternative therapist and some teachers will offer an introductory lesson free of charge. Teachers have completed an intensive three-year course approved by the international STAT organisation (Society of Teachers of the Alexander Technique).

CHIROPRACTIC

The name chiropractic originates from the Greek 'cheiro' meaning hand and 'praktos' meaning to use. It's the third largest healing profession worldwide, after medicine and dentistry, and is a manipulative therapy similar to osteopaihy, though in Britain there are many more qualified osteopaths than chiropractors and osteopathy is much better known.

So what are the differences between them? Both therapies were developed and first used towards the end of the last century but were founded on different philosophies. Chiropractors believed that symptoms stemmed from disorders in the nervous system, whereas osteopaths considered that a poor blood supply to the affected part was responsible. Nowadays these differences have faded and those that do exist are mainly of technique. For instance, chiropractors use x-rays five times more frequently than osteopaths to make a diagnosis and check on progress during treatment. Many chiropractors have x-ray machines on their premises.

Osteopathic treatment tends to include more soft-tissue techniques (various types of massage) and indirect rather than direct ways of adjusting (manipulating) the affected joints. The emphasis in chiropractic is on prevention and adjustment. However there are also many similarities in the methods used and neither treatment includes any form of surgery and very rarely drugs, which greatly enhances their appeal to many people.

Chiropractors believe that most problems occur because of misalignment – or 'subluxation' – of one or more of the vertebrae which, they say, can irritate, pinch or cause pressure on a nerve resulting in pain or symptoms. And since the spine is the body's primary form of support as well as the channel for the spinal cord and the nervous systems, back and spinal difficulties can lead to discomfort and pain in many other parts of the body. For example, pains in your leg can often be the result of a trapped nerve in your back.

Chiropractors and osteopaths aim to realign the bones and reduce nerve irritation mainly through adjustment (manipulation). According to the British

Chiropractic Association your body is a machine which has power sources, wiring, electricity and lubrication, etc. But, like machines, it also has a mechanical structure which can become damaged and that can, in many cases, be a relationship between the spinal column and headaches.

Chiropractors are trained to look for the spinal nerve stress – or vertebral subluxations – that lie behind many headaches, sometimes with the help of x-rays. Once this kind of spinal stress is identified, the chiropractor can use specific techniques to correct the condition. And once the spinal stress is freed – especially when it's in the cervical spine or neck – long-term relief from headaches and migraine can be achieved.

In suitable cases, therapists say that people of any age, including children, can benefit. At the first visit the practitioner will take a full medical history to look for any underlying causes for the symptoms.

A common anxiety when deciding whether to try manipulation, and a question I'm often asked, is 'Will it hurt?' The answer is, it may – but usually only briefly and often not at all. Much will depend on how long-standing the problem is and on the tenseness of the muscles – pain is less likely the more relaxed you are, so try not to resist the manipulation.

The techniques used will vary according to the person's age and physique. As each person is different, an individual treatment programme will be devised. Strength on the part of the therapist is not an important element – success depends on using a carefully controlled force, speed and depth of adjustment learnt over years of training.

Do be sure the chiropractor has the initials DC after his or her name. To become a chiropractor students must follow a four-year full-time course, resulting in a BSc degree in Chiropractic. This is followed by another year's postgraduate course at an established clinic before the student is allowed to apply for membership of the British Chiropractic Association.

Because of the treatment's individuality there is no average length of time for the course of treatment you may need, so don't forget to ask for an estimate of how much the treatment is going to cost so that you can budget for it.

OSTEOPATHY

Osteopaths are now enjoying a surge of popularity and acceptance. The treatment has been described as the most orthodox of the unorthodox therapies and even the Prince of Wales is among its many fans, as his presence at the publication of a recent report supporting osteopathy as a therapy confirms.

The General Council and Register of Osteopaths describes the treatment as the 'science of human mechanics' as it's concerned with the structural and mechanical problems of the body.

Osteopaths are keen to point out that the therapy is more than manipulation alone. They use a variety of techniques from soft-tissue massages, to stretching, as well as the high-velocity thrust that most people associate with osteopathy. Actually, this type of manipulation is a minor part of the treatment and some osteopaths rarely, if ever, use it.

Osteopathic treatment tends to be pleasant and relaxing and tailored to suit the needs of the individual concerned. That's why when you first visit an osteopath you will be thoroughly questioned about your medical history and, in particular when it comes to migraine, just how and when the symptoms first began.

The osteopath may also give you advice on posture,

diet, your lifestyle, or stress, particularly if any of these factors seem to aggravate or trigger your migraines.

Don't entrust yourself to an osteopath without first checking his or her qualifications – you can always phone the Osteopathic Information Service on 071 439 7177.

REFLEXOLOGY

The origins of reflexology can be traced back thousands of years and the technique is thought to have been used by the Ancient Egyptians. The art of foot reflexology today was established in the 1930s by an American therapist called Eunice Ingham. Some people believe that this method of treatment can be helpful in alleviating all manner of ailments, from bunions, headaches, insomnia, to vertigo, even high cholesterol and deafness. I have to admit, I'm not convinced it can work for many of these conditions – though I would support their 'cure' for headaches, for example.

Reflexology works on the understanding that there are areas, called reflex points, on the feet and also hands, that match up with each organ, gland and structure of the body – the sole of the foot is thought to represent a map of the body. The spine's reflex point is along the inside edge of both feet which is supposed to be similar in shape to that of the spine. The four arches of the spine – cervical, thoracic, lumbar and sacral – are reflected in the four arches of the feet.

A treatment of reflexology can last around thirty to forty minutes and is likely to involve a variety of massage techniques using the thumb and index finger in addition to a way of rotating the foot, called reflex rotation or pivot-point technique. The technique is a gentle one and many people find it quite pleasurable.

It's considered that the main benefit is its powers of relaxation, which can relieve stress and tension. It's also said to improve blood supply and to encourage the unblocking of nerve impulses.

SHIATSU

Shiatsu is a Japanese form of therapy meaning 'finger pressure', although it can be applied with other parts of the hand, even with elbows and knees. Apparently, some people who can't bear the thought of needles choose shiatsu instead of acupuncture because of this.

Shiatsu involves pressure on the acupuncture points so that the balance of the body's energy can be restored to promote good health. Like acupuncture there is a variety of shiatsu techniques all linked by a belief in the basic principle – that a vital force, Ki, flows through the body via channels called meridians. Pressure applied to points along the meridians is thought to have a similar effect to the needles of acupuncture. Shiatsu involves two main techniques, pressure and stretching.

The therapy, it is claimed, eases stress, stiffness and pain as well as improving movements and a person's flexibility. It's also thought to improve circulation, help rid the body of toxins and generally make you feel more relaxed – and you don't need to be ill or in pain to benefit from the technique. A session usually lasts an hour and a course of treatment may involve around five or more visits.

YOGA

Yoga has been practised in India for centuries as a means of maintaining mental and physical health by helping to release physical and mental tension. It can lead to good posture by teaching you to breathe properly and become flexible and supple while heightening awareness of each part of the body as you stretch as far as you can without risking injury.

Some people believe that yoga is undergoing a resurgence in interest and is even threatening to replace Jane Fonda and the like as the main type of relaxation class. It's said to be an excellent means of managing stress because it is so calming. As you think about what's happening to your physical self, you have less tension and tend to wipe out jumbled thoughts and emotions from your mind. But nevertheless, don't rush into things: if you start a yoga class, take things slowly but surely.

6: SELF-HELP TREATMENT

WHAT YOU CAN BUY

Over the counter, you can buy a variety of painkillers to help ease migraine. These can be used to treat pain resulting from a wide variety of symptoms – as well as headaches, they can soothe pain in neuralgia, colds and influenza and help reduce temperature, rheumatic pain, period pain, dental pain, back ache, muscular pain and sore throats. Some products you can buy in shops or supermarkets in soluble or tablet form – soluble painkillers are said to work more quickly because the active ingredient is absorbed into the bloodstream faster than solid tablets. But all of them are available at the pharmacy – the only shop where all medicines are kept or overseen by a professional pharmacist. He or she knows about and can advise on any of the medicines that are sold – or dispensed, when you hand in a doctor's prescription. Certain medicines can be supplied either on prescription or over the counter, and the over-the-counter price is sometimes cheaper than the prescription charge so it is worth asking your pharmacist's advice on this.

The products you can buy mainly contain aspirin, paracetamol or a combination of the two, sometimes with the addition of the stimulant caffeine. Some also have small quantities of codeine and dihydrocodeine. Others contain ibuprofen. If you are taking one kind of analgesic you should not take another within four hours – overdoses can be dangerous. And don't forget that paracetamol can be found in some cold cures. Read the labels carefully if you're taking other medicines.

Painkillers of this nature will often help ease migraine if you take them early enough, which is why many people don't even bother to go to see their doctor once he or she has made an initial diagnosis of migraine. If you're one of these people, remember that as soon as you experience sensations or symptoms of an imminent attack you should take your preferred remedy immediately. Ask your pharmacist about maximum doses and doses for children.

Anti-inflammatory medicines like aspirin and ibuprofen can prevent the release of prostaglandins (which pass on pain signals to the brain) and so are recommended for migraine – although paracetamol can help ease the pain of a headache, too.

One clinical trial suggested that taking aspirin every other day in a low dose (75 milligrams) was effective in helping prevent migraine attacks. And there's no doubt about it, aspirin is a wonder drug – new uses for it are constantly being discovered. For example, doctors usually recommend it to sufferers following a heart attack, to be taken in a similarly small dose to the one above, to help prevent further heart problems of a thrombotic kind – when the blood clots abnormally in an artery or vein. The effect it has is to prevent the blood's circulating platelet cells from sticking together too readily.

As I explained earlier, the platelets are nature's 'sandbags'. When a tear or injury occurs to blood vessels or tissues in the body, the local platelets start to stick together and jam into the hole, just like we push sandbags into a gap in a dam to prevent the water escaping. They stem the flow very quickly while the body starts to lay down fibres to 'cement' the platelets in place and a scar is quickly formed.

It is possible that this 'sticky' quality of the platelets increases the viscosity of the blood when the blood flow decreases in the early stages of a migraine and that this, in part, is responsible for some of the symptoms. It's possible that this is how a small dose of aspirin, by dampening the 'stickiness', is able to help prevent migraine (but don't take it regularly without consulting the doctor first).

Aspirin (available from chemists and supermarkets under 'own brand' labels) can irritate the stomach and if it's used for a long time can cause bleeding. That's why aspirin shouldn't be taken on an empty stomach, and at the very least with a glass of milk. Don't drink alcohol either when you're taking aspirin, it only adds to the likelihood of your stomach being irritated. Do not take aspirin if you have a stomach ulcer, and it is not usually recommended near the end of a pregnancy, either. Products helpful in easing a migraine headache containing aspirin include Anadin Extra (which contains aspirin, paracetamol and caffeine) and Anadin Maximum Strength (aspirin and caffeine); Aspro Clear; Codis 500 (aspirin and codeine phosphate); Disprin Direct (tablets containing aspirin which disperse on the tongue without water); Veganin (aspirin, paracetamol and codeine phosphate) and Powerin (aspirin, paracetamol and caffeine).

Another type of painkiller you can buy over the counter is codeine. This is a mild narcotic used in combination with paracetamol and sometimes aspirin. It blocks transmission of pain signals within the brain and the spinal cord. Don't take codeine-containing medicines if you are pregnant, or think you may be, as it has not been tested to prove that it is safe during pregnancy. However, don't be alarmed if you took a tablet or two before you knew you were pregnant, since it has not been specifically shown to *cause* any harm either.

Ibuprofen – widely available as Nurofen, Reclofen, Inoven and others – is, as I've said, an NSAID (non-steroidal anti-inflammatory drug, see page 54) which relieves pain, reduces inflammation and lowers temperature. It has been found in use to be gentler on the stomach than aspirin (though there is no obvious explanation for this as they work in similar ways) and as a result is tolerated just as well as aspirin.

Even so, it shouldn't be taken if you have a stomach ulcer or other stomach disorder. Asthma sufferers and anyone who is allergic to aspirin should only take ibuprofen after consulting their doctor. It's not suitable for pregnant women.

If you find paracetamol helpful you could try 'own brand' labels from chemists or supermarkets. Some examples of brand names available are: Anadin Paracetamol, Coda-Med (paracetamol, caffeine and codeine); Codanin (strong analgesic tablets containing paracetamol and codeine - uses include the relief of bad headaches and migraine); Disprin Extra (tablets containing aspirin and paracetamol); Disprol; Hedex; Panadeine (paracetamol and codeine phosphate); Panadol Extra (paracetamol and caffeine); Paraclear (soluble paracetamol); Paracodol (paracetamol and codeine phosphate); Solpadeine (paracetamol, codeine phosphate and caffeine); and Tramil 500.

There is a relatively new pain reliever available, called Paramol, containing the highly effective compound dihydrocodeine. This is one of the strongest pain-relieving compounds and until recently it has only been available on prescription. Paramol combines dihydrocodeine with the tried and trusted pain relief of paracetamol. As it is one of the strongest pain relievers you can buy, it must only be used as directed. If you suffer from asthma or have breathing difficulties, consult your doctor or pharmacist before taking Paramol.

There are also tablets available over the counter which are specially designed to relieve a migraine headache. These can contain analgesics combined with buclizine hydrochloride or cyclizine hydrochloride

– antihistamines to prevent vomiting and reduce nausea. Sufferers usually work out which treatment suits them best. Examples include Femigraine – soluble tablets containing aspirin to relieve migraine and cyclizine hydrochloride to help reduce vomiting and nausea. These tablets may cause drowsiness. Do not take them if you have a stomach ulcer or other stomach disorder, nor if you are sensitive to aspirin. Consult your doctor if you suffer from asthma, if you are receiving medical treatment or if you are pregnant.

Migraleve helps relieve migraine headache, nausea and vomiting. It's been specially designed to combine treatment for the symptoms of migraine while at the same time minimising the risk of side-effects. A pack contains eight pink and four yellow tablets. The pink tablets contain the pain-relievers paracetamol and codeine phosphate and the antihistamine buclizine hydrochloride. The yellow tablets do not contain the antihistamine.

When you take Migraleve, you should take two pink tablets at the first sign of a migraine attack. Or, if you experience migraine with aura, as soon as you experience your particular type of aura. Taking Migraleve immediately can prevent an attack.

It's important to take the tablets as soon as you feel a migraine developing because delay may allow the attack to get a hold so that any treatment might only be able to reduce the severity of the symptoms. If further treatment is needed, take two yellow tablets every four hours.

Some sufferers are able to tell when they're likely to get an attack, perhaps the day before their period, for example, or after an important examination. In cases like this, you could try taking two pink Migraleve either the night before, or a few hours prior to such a trigger. This can help prevent the attack.

Migraleve is not suitable for children under ten and can sometimes cause drowsiness. As with all medicines that might cause drowsiness, if affected don't drive or operate machinery and avoid alcoholic drink.

Propain (paracetamol, codeine phosphate and diphenhydramine hydrochloride and caffeine) shouldn't be taken during pregnancy or while breastfeeding. Also avoid excessive intake of coffee or tea when taking these tablets since propain contains caffeine and the extra intake in the drinks may keep you awake at night or make you feel 'on edge'. However, propain may also cause drowsiness since diphenhydramine is known to have sedative properties.

Nelsons, New Era and Weleda make a range of homoeopathic remedies which are widely available in health shops and even some chemists. Those suitable for migraine include, for example, Nelsons Classical Series *Kali. Bich.*, *Nat. Mur.*, *Nux. Vom*, New Era Migraine, Nervous Headaches and Weleda's Hom-Bidor 1%. (See also page 75 for more on homeopathy.)

Herbal remedies do seem to be increasing in popularity these days. But please be aware that just because a remedy has been used for hundreds of years, or just because it's 'natural' it doesn't necessarily mean it's OK. 'Natural' doesn't automatically mean 'harmless' or 'without side-effects', such as irritability or sleeplessness, for example. Potter's, Heath and Heather, and Gerard herbal products are popular and are available from health shops and some chemists. You could also try Herbal Laboratories Feverfew 125 and Golden Health Feverfew.

PREVENTION

If you think you are suffering from migraine, or experience one for the first time, consult your doctor for a proper diagnosis and advice on treatment. This will also reassure you that your migraines are not due to a tumour or to high blood pressure – two very common and usually quite unfounded fears, as I explained at the beginning of the book.

To help you and your doctor pinpoint your special triggers, try to keep a diary, or even a wall chart. Note the day and time of your attacks, everything you eat and drink, meal times, daily activities, particular worries and, for women, the dates of your periods. It's important to note down anything you might have done, even the slightest change of routine, for example, or whatever you might have eaten or drunk in the twelve to thirty-six hours that precede a migraine attack, no matter how trivial you might think it is. That kind of tiny detail could eventually emerge as a pattern over a length of time. And it's only when it's noted down that such a detail might strike you as being linked to your migraines. And by detail I also mean factors such as what the weather was like, what your mood was like, were you upset about something, whether or not you were constipated, etc.

But a word of advice here, don't pin too much on finding your trigger factors. I'd hate to give you false hope, although some sufferers have told me that just keeping a diary made them feel better because at last they were doing something to control their migraines. But remember, some people simply aren't able to work out what provokes their migraine – so if this happens to you, don't feel that yet again you are being singled out and that you must be the only one it doesn't work for. Many sufferers just have to accept that they'll never know their trigger factors.

Nevertheless, it is worth trying to find out. If you can work out what triggers your migraine, and therefore increase the likelihood of being able to avoid attacks, it is a better course of action than simply taking drugs to control them. Prevention is almost always better than cure. So to recap briefly, common trigger factors are food, drink, eating at irregular times or going without food (both of which contribute to a low blood sugar level), alcoholic drink, exercise, weather (be it thunder, sudden changes in the type of weather or temperature, or glaring sunlight), anxiety, stress, tension, shock and hormonal triggers such as menstrual periods.

But other events may also spark off an attack – common factors like the onset of hayfever, the common cold or toothache, or a change in prescription medicine. If you find they do then whenever such a provocation strikes it could be worthwhile instituting your own prevention (prophylactic) programme of the kind that was referred to on page 62.

But treatment as I've already said will depend on the frequency of attacks and the apparent causes. Simply adjusting your habits may help considerably and I can't repeat too often that any medicines should be taken at the first sign of an attack, so always keep them handy.

It also usually helps to rest quietly in a darkened room in the early stages. During a migraine, the action of the gut slows down and painkillers may not be well absorbed which is why some people find that soluble painkillers are more effective as they're said to be absorbed more quickly. Some of the medicines available from your doctor speed up absorption as well as relieving the nausea and pain. Other drugs act by constricting the dilated blood vessels, but follow the instructions precisely as overuse can actually bring on a headache similar to migraine.

As I've already explained, irregular meals, dieting or a long lie-in can provoke a migraine, probably because of the drop in the body's blood sugar. Then a few biscuits or a sweet drink may be enough to stave off a full attack. And if you can't go without your Saturday or

Sunday morning lie-in, why not take a snack to bed with you so you can eat something as soon as you wake without having to get out of bed!

It's extremely important to make sure you always eat properly and pay attention to your diet – not just at the weekend. If you think you'll have to go a long time without a proper meal, keep an emergency ration of a small snack of some sort with you. Skipping meals really isn't a good idea for a migraine sufferer.

Many sufferers say that nothing much helps ease the pain of an attack and all you can do is just live through it. But you could give some of the following self-help measures a try. Relieving the pain with a hot water bottle can help, so too can an ice pack. Some sufferers find that a cold shower concentrated on the head can ease the pain, and according to the Migraine Trust soaking your feet in hot water may be useful. It's likely that these straightforward measures work because they provide what's called a counter-irritant. The sensation of the cold water on the head, for example, sends impulses to the brain which takes its 'attention' away from the other painful impulses it's receiving. It's a bit like a switch-board operator being less angry with an obnoxious caller if the switchboard is jammed with other irate callers – she is more inclined to shrug her shoulders and see Mr Obnoxious for what he is, and so not let it 'get to her'.

One sufferer tells me that when she has to lie in a dark room to overcome her migraine attack, she does find that cold flannels over her forehead are helpful in slightly easing the pain. Another suggests buying a soothing eye mask from the Body Shop. The gel-filled mask costs £5.50 and is called a Soothe Pack. It can be used either cold or hot, whichever temperature you find most comforting. It's up to you to try these different options and work out which one is best for you.

Wearing dark glasses often relieves the pain of a headache slightly, especially if you are one of the many sufferers who dislike brightness during an attack.

I'm quite convinced that VDUs worry a great many sufferers. I'm regularly asked whether they can aggravate migraine. Well, the answer is yes. Many sufferers do insist that working with a computer screen triggers an attack. My advice is to make sure that you do not sit at the screen all day long. If you can't mix your work schedule to involve intervals away from it, then do ensure you take short, regular breaks. Also, try to position your screen in such a way as to avoid glare or reflections.

When migraine does strike, don't try to soldier on regardless. It's best to stop what you are doing and, if you are at work, try to go home to sleep. So many sufferers try to carry on in the hope that they'll work through the attack, but more often than not this just prolongs the agony. And most of the time they end up having to go to bed anyway.

Although for some people sleep (especially too much of it) can trigger a migraine, generally speaking it does have a positive effect during an attack and helps many sufferers – that is, if they are able to go to sleep. The amount of sleep needed varies from person to person: some find they need only a short nap to get some relief, while others need a really good sleep of up to several hours. That's why if you wake with a migraine, you should take medication as soon as you can, and then stay in bed.

As I've said, sleep is beneficial for migraine, but some sufferers find that sleeping in the wrong type of atmosphere can be a trigger for an attack. Albert who spoke about his 'bilious attacks' on page 50, believes that he is a 'headachy' person. In other words, he believes he has a headache waiting to 'come out' all the time. When a headache has developed, he cannot tolerate being in a hot room.

> I find it's much better to lie down in a dark, cool room. Even if I don't have a migraine and sleep in a room that's stuffy – usually centrally heated – I can wake with a headache.

Climate and the weather seem to affect migraine sufferers. Many people find that they get a headache when they are out in a cold wind. The pain here is likely to be due to muscular tension in the scalp or the blood vessels in the head. When the cold causes the small blood vessels to constrict – so cooling the skin to prevent heat loss from the body – the muscles overdo it a bit in susceptible areas. The muscles close by also go into spasm in a reflex action.

I've found that this can be prevented in some people if the ears are covered, so if you don't do so already, make sure that you wear a head scarf, ear muffs or hat which comes down over your ears.

Also some sufferers claim that a small electric ioniser can bring benefits, either preventing migraines or reducing their frequency. The theory behind this is that it corrects the balance of the electrical charges in the air – the ions. I'm not convinced. If you know a friend who has one (often stored in their loft since they no longer use it!) why don't you ask if you can borrow it and see if it works for you. It certainly can't do any harm and I'm a great believer in giving anything that doesn't do any harm – and that you can afford – a try (before it goes back in the loft!).

Another sufferer told me that she found that a migraine came on after she defrosted the freezer.

> I don't know whether it was the combination of cold air and my bending down, but I had such a bad migraine, I've

never defrosted the freezer since. Now my husband does it. I've found it helps if I can work out something that triggers an attack, and if my husband can easily do the job instead of me, that's what we'll do.

If you're sensitive to smells, particularly perfume, don't wear it – it's better to be safe than sorry. Or take the advice of one sufferer – if you sit next to someone on a train or bus who's wearing strong perfume, don't be embarrassed, or sit there hoping you'll get away with it, just get up and move to another seat. Remember, getting a migraine is worse than the few moments it takes to change seats.

And the same applies to smoking. Though if, as is likely, you're already in a no-smoking compartment and someone is just being bad-mannered, again it's better just to move away than start a punch-up with the possibility of also starting – at best! – another migraine.

Going on holiday seems to be a frequent trigger factor for many people, obviously with the build up of pressure – trying to finish lots of work before you go, or the pressures of getting a family ready for the off. It's probably helpful to try to get as organised as you can as far in advance as possible. Slow but sure planning is far better than leaving everything to the last minute so that it's one big stressful rush. And while you're on holiday don't forget that you still need to be careful about avoiding your trigger factors.

Sheila, a twenty-six-year-old single parent and part-time domestic cleaner, believes that overdoing things is a sure way to provoke a migraine. And she says it's also important to remember not to dash around and start doing lots of things when you've just got over an attack.

My migraines have been so bad that I have to lie in a very dark room, sometimes for three days. I could be sick about twenty times a day, which is really unpleasant. I can't stand anyone to move the bed or to touch me. If during that time anyone asked me my phone number, I wouldn't even be able to remember it.

Being a single parent has made life difficult at times, and has prompted Sheila to find lots of ways of coping with an attack.

My daughter used to be frightened of my migraines. She told her teacher that I'd had a heart attack – that was the only way she could explain the awful thing that was happening to me. Yet at five years old I had to teach her how to use the phone, most importantly to ring her father, from whom I'm divorced. At six, she used to empty sick bowls because I couldn't get out of bed to do it. While I'm ill she's as good as gold. But when I'm better her fear seems to come out and she'll cry. Children have to grow up so quickly when a parent is ill.

Now I do find that it definitely helps me to try to have a rest every day when my daughter is at school. I go to bed for an hour and a half. Even if I don't manage to sleep at all, I do unwind. I also make sure that I go to bed at ten o'clock every night. The other day I was out at a wedding and I didn't get to bed until about one o'clock in the morning. And sure enough I got a migraine the next day.

Sometimes it can take me a week to get over an attack because I find it impossible to sleep, so I'm physically exhausted but mentally so pleased it's over. When the pain has gone it's like winning the pools. My first reaction is to go out, perhaps to the shops because I'm so pleased I'm able to do it, but when you're not really fit after getting over an attack, that's when you're likely to trigger off another one. You do need to be careful not to overdo things.

Many people are reluctant to join a support group, but it can be extremely beneficial for all manner of problems – not least because it so often dispels feelings of isolation. Sheila believes that joining the British Migraine Association was a definite step in the right direction.

> Another thing I've found helpful is becoming a member of the British Migraine Association. When I first had migraine I didn't know anyone else with it. So when I received the association's newsletter for the first time, I sat down and cried because I thought, at last, I feel as if I'm not alone. Knowing you're not on your own does help.

Sheila is one of the many migraine sufferers who has found the new drug, Imigran, helpful, although she feels it does tend only to suppress the pain that will eventually find its way out. But she has also tried a variety of other measures to cope with her attacks. She has even tried spiritual healing which she found beneficial because it helped her achieve inner strength.

> The healer counselled me about trying to be strong in myself. I'm a very placid, calm person and I've found that being near loud, aggressive people upsets me. Learning to cope with that helps. Another way spiritual healing has helped me is if I'm feeling tired and someone rings at the door wanting a two-hour chinwag I'm now strong enough to say I'm sorry I can't talk at the moment I need a rest.

Many people find that they feel very calm and relaxed after visiting a healer. The usual format is that the sufferer sits in a chair with their feet firmly on the ground. You relax, shut your eyes and the healer holds his or her hands over the crown of your head. Some people feel sensations of heat or cold, tingling, or pins and needles. The healing process is said to go through the healer to you. Some people explain it as universal energy, some believe it's God. In my opinion, whatever the explanation, if it brings any relief it's to be welcomed. Make sure the healer is 'recognised' and not a charlatan, and that he or she charges a reasonable rate. Many healers won't accept a fee, perhaps believing that their powers are God-given.

Meditation is another skill Sheila has learned to her benefit.

> If you can make a time each day, say half an hour before bed, it is a really good way of getting the day's events off your mind. I also try to meditate at lunchtime when I'm resting. I try to focus on a relaxing scene, perhaps sitting by a lake, watching the water. If the water is rough I try to calm it down in my mind, or if I'm sitting by a rough sea I try to calm the waves. When I first tried it, I thought I wouldn't possibly be able to do it or concentrate enough, but with a bit of practice it becomes easier.

Relaxation techniques can be useful in coping with pain, but can also help by reducing tension and stress which may be triggers of your migraine. Pain can make you anxious which in turn makes you tense your muscles, tugging on the joints and adding to your discomfort. You can easily become trapped in a vicious circle of pain, then tension, then more pain.

When it comes to relaxation techniques, it does help if you choose half an hour or so when you're likely to be undisturbed. Another useful pointer when starting out is to try to have a bed or sofa to lie on, and to try to make sure the room you use is comfortably warm and peaceful.

It can take a while before you get the hang of the technique – you may even need to give it a go every day for a month. But once perfected you'll probably find it won't matter where you are. And you can spend as long as you think you need to relax totally.

You learn to relax by resting with your arms and legs unfolded and uncrossed. Think about the way you are breathing and try to breathe slowly and regularly.

Focus on your muscles, tense them or imagine that they are becoming very heavy. Or, you can concentrate on different parts of your body, working down from your head to your toes. When you release your muscles, let them go as much as possible. It helps, too, if you take long, slow breaths, and try to think about nothing else or, if you can't clear your mind, at least think of something pleasant!

I find that if I'm trying to relax and my mind is spinning with endless thoughts, I concentrate on one meaningless word and exclude all other thoughts which helps keep my attention focused on what's happening to my body.

Carrying out a quick facial relaxation is also useful. Muscles in the face and neck are often responsible for headaches, neck and back pain. Try clenching the teeth and frowning heavily and feeling the whole of the face and neck tense up. Then let your jaw relax and your frown disappear and note how different this feels.

I tend to have tension in my shoulders and jaw, so I let my mouth fall wide open and then close it slightly, hunch my shoulders in an exaggerated fashion then let them relax. I stretch my hands and fingers like a fan and then relax them. The muscles of my forehead, too, are prone to be bunched and the skin crinkled into care lines, so I open my eyes wide, lift my brow then let the forehead relax back to where it was. As well as relaxation, hypnotherapy – which in a way is a form of deep relaxation – may be useful if you find that your migraines are related to stress or anxiety. Ideally the hypnotherapist should be recommended by your doctor since there are various hypnotherapy qualifying bodies but not one that is recognised in the same way as a medical or dental qualification. Indeed, your doctor may practise hypnotherapy – or may know of another doctor who does.

And if you find your migraine is getting you down, don't feel ashamed to have a good cry now and then. Give yourself permission to feel misery, resentment or even despair. You're not a wimp, crying releases the body's endorphins, those natural salves of pain, both physical and emotional. Sometimes a good cry probably has as much benefit as a prescription. Laughing, too, is also a good relaxation treatment. It reduces muscular tension, improves breathing, regulates the heart beat and pumps adrenaline and endorphins into the bloodstream.

Exercise can be helpful in cutting down migraine attacks and aid their prevention. It helps you lose weight, keeps you in trim, strengthens your muscles and so increases your stamina, and helps maintain a healthy heart. It improves your suppleness and is a good way of working stress out of your system – which is definitely beneficial for anyone who knows that stress can trigger an attack. And remember, exercise can be something as simple as going for a brisk walk. Swimming is very good for relaxing, and if you're not a good swimmer, don't worry, it helps even if you just swim a width of the pool. The next time you go you'll be able to do a little more. Cycling is good and gentle jogging can be beneficial, though best done with good-quality shock-absorbing shoes and on grass rather than hard roads.

But before you rush to pull on your jogging shoes, do remember that even exercise has been known to trigger migraines. Short, sharp shocks to the system, particularly when you're not especially fit or not used to exercising, can reduce blood sugar levels which may then lead to an attack.

When you exercise, your muscles need more blood so the blood vessels widen, especially those just under the skin, as witnessed by the flushed faces. The blood pressure also rises and this combination causes further stretching of the already dilated – opened – blood vessels inside the skull, which may cause a headache.

So if you want to exercise as a means of relaxation and achieving a higher level of fitness, do start off slowly but surely – little and often is the key.

Also, according to the Migraine Trust, a headache associated with sexual intercourse is an example of an exercise headache. It can happen at, or very near, the time of orgasm and can be quite severe, sometimes persisting for days, although it usually goes off quite soon. Women as well as men are affected. And, says the Trust, since the blood pressure can rise more than 50 per cent and the pulse rate double during intercourse, it is surprising that this type of headache is not more common. But though this may be a form of exercise headache, you should ignore the advice given in the previous paragraph – slowly but surely and little and often may be good for exercise in general, but it could wreak havoc in your sex life!

I've heard it said that a recommended daily allowance (known as an RDA) of Pyridoxine – Vitamin B6 – can help prevent an orgasmic headache. Though I know of no definite scientific evidence to support that, if you can afford it and stick to the RDA, what have you got to lose?

And such simple remedies do often work wonders. A migraine sufferer I know regularly played rugby and trained at his club twice each week. He often developed a migraine after a particularly vigorous game on a Saturday afternoon. This had usually been preceded by a long lie-in that morning. I suggested he chew some glucose tablets before a game, and a couple more at half-time, as well as making sure that he eat something, even if only a snack or sandwich, as soon as possible after showering and changing. This advice seemed to do the trick.

So when exercising make sure you eat a snack before

and after, and one that contains carbohydrate and protein so that it's absorbed slowly into the blood. A light meal of, for example, wholegrain rice or pasta flavoured with fish, meat or low-fat cheese will do nicely, as will a wholemeal bread sandwich with a fish, meat or low-fat cheese filling. Sweet foods, such as chocolate or sweets, are second best because they can cause a sudden surge in blood sugar levels which can then fall just as suddenly.

If you regularly feel stiffness or a tautness in your neck, shoulders and upper back at the end of a hard day's work, a combination of relaxation and exercise could be the thing for you, particularly if you feel this tension triggers your migraine. There's nothing quite like stress for causing muscle tension. When you feel yourself knotting up, work your way up or down your body, tensing and then relaxing your muscles as you go. Slow deep breathing, while thinking about those breaths, can also calm the nerves and tension.

DEALING WITH STRESS

Dealing with stress could be another way of controlling your migraines, especially if you know you are likely to develop one because of a stressful situation. If you're not aware of a particular situation causing you stress, then try looking at your life as if you were a fly on the wall. Very often it's easy to do this while you're on holiday – it's always easier to get things into perspective when you're out of your normal everyday situation and routines. Things might become clearer to you – whether it's realising how much you are worrying about your financial situation, or how boring you are finding your job, or thinking about where relationships are falling down, or whether it's simply that you are a very busy mother with little time to yourself. Try to work out compromises where you can. Allow time for yourself.

On a personal level, I find that I am quite a committed workaholic. But over the years I've discovered that giving myself time to regain a balance actually helps me work more effectively. I'm careful to exercise regularly, spend time with my family, my pets, in my garden, and sometimes just giving myself permission to sit quietly helps me relax.

Exercise and yoga are, or course, good ways to deal with stress. Another remedy may be aromatherapy. Aromatherapy is said to be relaxing and, as such, is ideal for treating stress and building up a resistance to it. It's also an excellent way of indulging yourself and allowing time *just for you*.

The process involves using powerful, natural plant essences derived from flowers, leaves, stems, roots or bark. They can be used in massage, added to your bath water or inhaled by adding a few drops to a bowl of hot water. You can either consult a professional aromatherapist or you can buy essential oils from health shops, pharmacists and the Body Shop. Nelson & Russell make a range of oils – for example, their Ylang Ylang and Orange Bath and Massage Oils are said to be good for resting and relaxing. The Body Shop's rose or lavender oils are also recommended for relaxation – lavender helps relieve tension-related problems and rose is said to be soothing for nervous and premenstrual tension. Other oils that can help induce a feeling of well-being are rosewood, frankincense and clary sage. When you need uplifting you could try lemon, rosemary or sandalwood.

But a word of warning – neat essential oils shouldn't be used directly on the skin, they should be diluted in a 'carrier' oil. And some aromatherapy oils should not be used if you are pregnant or suffer from epilepsy or other conditions. Don't leave the tops off containers, as the oils are highly volatile and can soon evaporate. Keep them well away from children and never use them near the eyes. Do not take them internally either. Some migraine sufferers find aromatherapy a helpful means of relaxation, but others, who are sensitive to smells, may not find this treatment particularly helpful.

Massage, too, is thought to be excellent for relaxation. Massaging the body's soft tissue, its muscles and ligaments can encourage calm sensations. It doesn't have to be relaxing either – it can also be invigorating, depending on the kind of massage you choose.

Another way of relieving stress, which is probably one of the most inexpensive ways of doing it, is talking about something that might be worrying you. Talk to a friend, a colleague or a member of your family. Sometimes a simple chat with someone can help put a stressful situation into perspective – as the saying goes 'A problem shared is a problem halved.' Talking is so straightforward and yet it's not always as uncomplicated as it could be. It can be difficult if we dread what others will think of what we have to say. My advice is always: if you value the person you're with and are confident of them, it's worth the risk. Seeking help isn't a sign of weakness. I believe it's a sign of strength to overcome the temptation to bottle up your feelings and to allow yourself to look for and accept care and advice from others.

MIGRAINE AND WORK

Work can become impossible for many a migraine sufferer. If you have frequent migraines you can become a victim of unsympathetic employers and resentful colleagues who might think you are taking excess time off with a feeble excuse. One sufferer has even recently received her first verbal warning at work due to absences relating to migraine. Another told me she definitely lost one high-powered job because of it.

Anne, who discussed her beneficial experience with Imigran on page 58, was secretary to a company managing director and was on a six-month trial period. At the end of the six months her employment was terminated – and migraine, not any complaints about the standard of her work, was given as the reason.

> The job was quite stressful and I did have more migraines than I normally would have. At the worst point, I was having one every ten days. I have to say that I did find another job soon after that that wasn't quite as stressful and I did have a boss who told me not to worry about my migraines. As a result I wasn't under so much stress and my migraine attacks became less frequent. So I'm one of the lucky ones.

If your work is causing extra stress, and the hints given on page 103 aren't helping, your choices are several. If the firm is a medium to large one it could have an occupational health service, so make an appointment to see the nurse or doctor. Either will be well versed in stress and its management. They are also well placed to have a discreet word with senior managers if they consider that the tasks or pressures expected of you are unreasonable.

If such a service isn't available, have a word with your boss, if he or she is the kind of individual who will understand and listen. If they're not, your choices are starker. You could try to soldier on, in the hope that things will get better, especially if the work is seasonal or cyclical. You could see if there is a way to delegate some of your work or responsibilities, or you could find another job if that is a good possibility. Whichever course you choose, good luck.

CHARLOTTE: A CASE STUDY

For Charlotte, a twenty-two-year-old secretary, accepting that she has migraine and truly believing that there is nothing 'wrong' with her, has been one of the major breakthroughs she has made in coping with the condition. For her the problem has frequently been severe and totally debilitating. Attacks as often as two or three times a week have meant that she could just about manage to carry out her job, go home, sleep and little else. Her lack of a social life and consequent loneliness at times drove her to thoughts of suicide and she even had to take anti-depressants for six months under the careful guidance of her GP.

She has suffered from migraine for the past seven years – although she didn't discover it was actually migraine until five years ago.

At first I seemed to have a constant headache every day. It felt as if my jaw was wired up all the time – as if I was clenching my teeth all the while without realising I was doing it. I had no idea then that it could be migraine, after all I didn't know much about it and didn't know anyone who suffered from it either. My doctor told me it was muscle tension at first.

Then the migraines got worse after about two years. They would last for a week and often I would feel awful and exhausted for the following week. I don't get visual disturbances, I just feel sick. Sometimes I get a horrible taste in my mouth and I know that there's nothing I can do to stop the attack coming. I almost wish then that it would hurry up and come so that I can get it over with. I also get a strange feeling, too, which is really hard to describe. It's like a tension headache but I know that it's simply building up to something much worse.

The pain is often so bad that sometimes I knock my head against a wall to distract my attention from the migraine. Whatever side of my head is aching I press really hard against the wall.

Charlotte has no idea what triggers her migraines. In the past she has dutifully kept a diary.

Anything could give me a migraine. I feel it could be linked to my menstrual cycle because I usually have an attack a week before my period, but then I have migraines at other times of the month, too. Staying up late definitely gives me one, or if I don't eat.

If I go to a disco, or a party, I always wake up the next morning with a migraine. I don't know whether it's the noise, or cigarette smoke, or the darkness, that brings it on.

She's tried all manner of things from conventional over-the-counter treatments, like Migraleve, to the new prescription medicine, Imigran, all without much success. In her desperate quest for relief she's tried quite a variety of alternative treatments, too.

I've even had a brain scan to establish that I didn't have a serious underlying condition. I wasn't really frightened by that. Of course, I was concerned, but I almost hoped that doctors would find something because then at least whatever it was could be treated and I would have a reason for suffering the way I was. I know that's a drastic reaction but that's how I felt about it.

I've tried feverfew every day for about four months. That was on the suggestion of my doctor who also suffers from migraine and finds that it works for her. That had no effect whatsoever.

I've tried acupuncture for about the same length of time, about two or three times a week. I had needles in my back, feet, in my head at the top and at the back of my neck, in my temples, in my legs. Each time it was somewhere different. The acupuncturist spent a lot of time talking to me as well. I'd often end up being there three hours at a time. I found it hard to relax, even though acupuncture is thought to help you do that. But it was good to talk to someone, to get my feelings off my chest.

For six months I had to take anti-depressants – that was two years ago. I struggled to go to work. I didn't ever go out. I had no social life. I was reluctant to make plans – it makes you even more depressed when you always have to cancel them because of your migraine. Then when you do feel well enough to go out, there's nobody there to go with. My family were supportive and did try to cheer me up but I just wanted to commit suicide.

I even went to see a psychologist at the beginning of last year. I also started to get panic attacks out of fear that I would have a migraine if I had to go into a meeting at work to take notes, or if I had to go out. I'd sit at my desk and feel so faint that I had to hold on to something, or I would just have to run out of the office, or I would feel really light-headed. I'd also panic that everyone was looking at me, or feel as if I had gone bright red.

Then it got so bad that sometimes I would have about four panic attacks a day, even when I wasn't thinking about something that might make me panic. I might be standing in a queue in a shop and it would just creep up. I'd either have to stick it out and quickly pay for what I wanted, or put the thing back on the shelf and leave the shop as quickly as I could.

I did find the psychologist helpful. I didn't think she would be when I first went. But I have been so desperate at times, I will keep trying anything. I had to record what I was thinking and what I was doing when I had a panic attack. She then set me goals, such as just planning one thing to do at the weekend instead of doing nothing. I joined a health club and aimed to go swimming at the weekend. She also taught me breathing exercises and re-assured me that nothing awful was going to happen to me.

Charlotte saw her psychologist monthly for six months and feels that it did help a great deal.

> I stopped going to her when I got to the stage where I felt I could cope. It was worthwhile because now I don't get the panic attacks so often and I can understand what is happening to my body.

Indeed, Charlotte is quite correct in saying that understanding what is happening to your body is useful in controlling panic attacks.

Nearly all of us have times when life puts terrific pressure on us, not just becoming very frightened that a migraine attack might interrupt our routine yet again. We may find it difficult to pay our mortgage, a relationship may be about to break up, or someone we love may be ill. Such events can often give us 'butterflies' in our stomach, funny sensations in our arms or legs, or make us feel sick and dizzy.

These unpleasant feelings are, in fact, mild panic attacks, though many people hesitate to pin such a big label on them. But in between the minor episodes of upsetting, panicky feelings there are a whole range of symptoms such as breathlessness, sweating, shaking, a fear that you're going to faint, or that your legs are about to collapse underneath you.

All of these symptoms are due to muscular tension in the body and a state of anxiety in the mind which literally knocks the body off balance physically, mentally and chemically.

Most of us find we can cope with periods of momentary unsteadiness, but when the condition begins to get as bad as it did for Charlotte, with attacks coming as often as four times a day, then it's understandable that the help of a clinical psychologist should be sought. Like Charlotte, most people react against this advice initially and don't quite believe that it's going to help, but they soon realise and accept that the cure lies within themselves.

Many former sufferers have told me that, once they allowed themselves to experience their fears through a full panic attack, from a position of safety, they were surprised to find that the world didn't swallow them up as they had believed. In this way, they begin to rid themselves of the 'fear of the fear' that haunts them. If you find you suffer from panic attacks because of the worry of getting a migraine, please remember these attacks don't cease immediately. You may have to go through the experience again several times. However, the symptoms lessen in severity each time and, gradually, the fear that accompanies them is reduced until the vicious circle is broken. Many sufferers in their teens and twenties, who have managed to overcome the problem of panic attacks, find it hard to believe that the experience actually happened to them – even though it made such an enormous impact on their lives at the time.

But Charlotte's quest for help didn't stop at the psychologist. She's tried hypnotherapy, spiritual healing and tests for food allergies.

I began to feel desperate to find a cure for my migraines and tried ten weeks of hypnotherapy – I'm always keen to try out ideas that anyone suggests to me.

The hypnotherapist would try to relax me by suggesting I imagine I was somewhere I liked – by the beach, for example – and then helped me become more relaxed. She questioned why I thought I had a headache, but I felt that she was trying to delve into my past for a reason for my headaches, such as the fact that my parents split up when I was four years old – reasons that I didn't believe were there. The sessions just annoyed me and I didn't feel they helped at all. Spiritual healing didn't help much either.

Nor did going to an allergy centre. The only thing I found I was allergic to was cats and dogs – which doesn't give you migraine anyway. I tried a diet of lamb and pears for seven days and only drank water – and I had the most terrible migraines during that week! I've had a tooth out at the dentist to see whether that would help. I've kept a diary for two years to try to see what triggers the migraines. All to no avail.

When patients are put on 'elimination' diets, so to speak, they are usually restricted to foods such as lamb, pears, fish, carrots and mineral water. These foods are selected because they are unlikely to cause symptoms of allergy. A single food is then introduced, so working out exactly what food could be a trigger. This kind of treatment is no good for those without patience as it can take as long as six to eight weeks to test foods. I really feel that this type of treatment should be carried out under medical supervision. Many sufferers, from conditions where food allergies may play a part, are increasingly turning to elimination diets to 'cure' their symptoms, and are sometimes following them for months if not for years. Nutritional deficiency syndromes have, in the past, been an all too tragic consequence of drought or starvation. It would be equally tragic if such states occurred in the developed world as the side-effect of such treatments.

Having tried so many alternative treatments, Charlotte looked forward to the arrival of a new conventional medicine, Imigran. But once again she was to be disappointed.

I was really excited about trying Imigran, but that didn't work for me either, in fact I felt worse. And then on top of that I was really disappointed and felt singled out yet again.

Now I tend not to say anything to anyone when I have a migraine just in case I feel even worse the next day. These days I keep it to myself as much as I can. My boss isn't very sensitive and when I have had to have time off because of a migraine I am sure that he thinks I've been out and have just got a hangover. I think that's because so often people who don't suffer from migraine use it as an excuse to have a day off – that's why I'd rather not say anything about it.

If I need to stay in bed I put a limit on myself as to how long I stay there. If it's a Saturday morning I will make myself get up at twelve, unless the migraine is so bad I can hardly stand, even if it's to do one thing like the dusting, or just to go out for half an hour. I find making myself keep going helps.

These days I feel as if I am in control of my migraines more. Just accepting it has helped. I appreciate now that it's not curable but I can control it by all sorts of self-help measures, such as eating regularly, taking painkillers as soon as I feel an attack coming on, as well as other types of medication. I wish when I first found out that I had migraine someone had just explained this to me. I could have accepted it much earlier and learned to live with it instead of constantly worrying that there was something 'wrong' with me and desperately seeking a cure.

Charlotte has discovered, for herself, what works best for her. But I wonder if she would have felt in control, as she does now, if she had had an explanation but hadn't tried all the possibilities. I doubt it, but we can't be sure.

I believe it depends very much on the individual's personality as to how they reach their goal. If my migraine had persisted I think that, like her, I would have tried every responsible preventive and treatment regime.

My hope is that this book may give you the explanation you need, and inspire the will that Charlotte had to get it under control.

HELPFUL ADDRESSES

UNITED KINGDOM

British Chiropractic Association,
29 Whitley Street, Reading, Berkshire RG2 OEG.
Tel: 0734 757557.

The association maintains a register of all qualified chiropractors in membership, which is limited exclusively to graduates of recognised chiropractic colleges. The Anglo-European College of Chiropractic and the colleges affiliated to the Council on Chiropractic Education, the government-recognised accrediting agency for chiropractic education in the United States, are the colleges recognised by the association.

The register of members is published to provide the public with the names of chiropractors whose training and ethical conduct can be relied upon. All these chiropractors have graduated with the following qualifications: DC, B.App. Sc(Chiro), BSc Chiropractic or BSc Chiropractic DC. For a copy of the register and further information contact the association.

British Homoeopathic Association,
27a Devonshire Street, London W1N 1RJ.
Tel: 071 935 2163.

For books, advice, information and a list of practitioners.

British Migraine Association, 178A High Road, Byfleet, West Byfleet, Surrey, KT14 7ED.
Tel: 0932 352468.

The association was set up in 1958, by a small group of migraine sufferers. It's still run for sufferers by sufferers, their families and friends. It raises money for research and publishes educational leaflets which are free to members. Some members have taken part in research experiments and drug trials.

Council for Acupuncture, 179 Gloucester Place, London NW1 6DX. Tel: 071 724 5756.
Send £2.50 and an A5 addressed envelope for a directory of British acupuncturists.

General Council and Register of Osteopaths, 56 London Street, Reading, Berkshire RG1 4SQ. Tel: 0734 576585
For names and addresses of registered osteopaths in your area.

Institute for Complementary Medicine, PO Box 194, London SE16 1QZ. Tel: 071 237 5165.
Send a large SAE with three loose stamps and a clear indication of what kind of information you'd like and on what subject. The institute holds the British register of complementary practitioners and can also give advice on training and courses.

MIGRAINE CLINICS

The City of London Migraine Clinic, 22 Charterhouse Square, London EC1M 6DX.
Will also treat patients without an appointment during an acute attack. This clinic is a charity and donations are gratefully received.

Princess Margaret Migraine Clinic, Charing Cross
Hospital, Fulham Palace Road, London W6 8RF.
Will also treat patients during acute attacks. A National
Health Service clinic.

The Migraine Trust, 45 Great Ormond Street,
London, WC1N 3HD.

The trust funds research and clinics, holds international symposia and provides help and information
for sufferers. Since its formation in 1965, it has funded
some of the major advances in migraine research in the
world. For example, it's already planning a Brain Bank
so that scientists can analyse the essential difference
between migraine sufferers and normal subjects.

Every second year, the trust holds an international
symposium in London attended by neurologists, other
specialists and scientists working in the field of
migraine. This world-leading symposium is attended by
more than one thousand delegates from fifty countries.

The trust also helps fund migraine clinics throughout
the country and encourages the formation of self-help
groups.

For an up-to-date list of clinics as well as hospitals
with particular interest in migraine you can contact The
Migraine Trust Helpline on 071 278 2676.

Osteopathic Information Service.
Tel: 071 439 7177.

**Society of Teachers of the Alexander Technique
(STAT)**, 20 London House, 266 Fulham Road,
London SW10 9EL. Tel: 071 351 0828.

For more information or a list of around six hundred
specialist teachers who have taken a three-year training
course approved by the society, you can write to STAT
enclosing an SAE.

AUSTRALIA

AFONTA (Australian Federation of Natural Therapy Associations), 8 Thorp Road, Woronora, New South Wales 2232. Tel: 02 521 2063.

Australasian Council on Chiropractic and Osteopathic Education Ltd, 941 Neopean Highway, Mornington, Victoria 3931. Tel: 059 75 35 46.

Australian Osteopathic Association, 2 Hillside Parade, Gleniris 3146. Tel: 03 889 6765.

CANADA

The Migraine Foundation, 120 Carlton Street, Suite 210, Toronto, Ontario M5A 4K2. Tel: 416 920 4916.

INDEX